100 Questions & Answers About Metastatic Breast Cancer

Lillie D. Shockney, RN, BS, MAS, HON-ONN-CG

Former Director
Johns Hopkins Breast Center
University Distinguished Service Professor of Breast Cancer
Professor of Surgery
Johns Hopkins University School of Medicine
Baltimore, Maryland

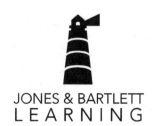

JONES & BARTLETT
LEARNING

World Headquarters
Jones & Bartlett Learning
5 Wall Street
Burlington, MA 01803
978-443-5000
info@jblearning.com
www.jblearning.com

Jones & Bartlett Learning books and products are available through most bookstores and online booksellers. To contact Jones & Bartlett Learning directly, call 800-832-0034, fax 978-443-8000, or visit our website, www .jblearning.com.

Substantial discounts on bulk quantities of Jones & Bartlett Learning publications are available to corporations, professional associations, and other qualified organizations. For details and specific discount information, contact the special sales department at Jones & Bartlett Learning via the above contact information or send an email to specialsales@jblearning.com.

Production Credits

VP, Product Development: Christine Emerton
Director of Product Management: Matt Kane
Product Manager: Joanna Gallant
Content Strategist: Christina Freitas
Content Strategist: Melina Leon
Project Manager: Kristen Rogers
Senior Project Specialist: Dan Stone
Senior Digital Project Specialist: Angela Dooley

Marketing Manager: Lindsay White
Product Fulfillment Manager: Wendy Kilborn
Composition: S4Carlisle Publishing Services
Text Design: Kristin E. Parker
Cover Design: Scott Moden
Cover Image: © SDI Productions/Getty images
Printing and Binding: CJK Group Inc.

ISBN: 978-1-284-22071-1

6048

Printed in the United States of America
25 24 23 22 21   10 9 8 7 6 5 4 3 2 1

Contents

Part 5: Hormonal Therapy   63

Part 6: HER2–Positive Biologic Targeted Therapy   77

Part 7: Side Effects of Metastatic Breast Cancer and Its Treatment

Foreword

Breast cancer remains the most feared disease among women. Receiving a diagnosis of stage IV breast cancer is a shock, and it affects you and everyone who loves you. This book is designed to help you, and those who care about you, understand what metastatic breast cancer is and what treatment options there are. It will also help you make decisions regarding those treatment choices and help you plan for your future.

There are no magic bullets regarding treatment for this stage of disease. There is hope, and with more research being completed every year, that hope grows. Just in the past few years, wonderful progress has been made in the development of new drugs for metastatic breast cancer treatment and even new drug classifications than we had in the past.

There is also a better understanding of the feelings of isolation and misunderstanding that someone like you with metastatic breast cancer is experiencing and efforts to change those myths the general public has about metastatic breast cancer and support you so you don't feel like you're alone.

This book contains the top 100 questions women ask to help them understand their disease, how best to decide what treatments will be right for each patient, and other matters that impact their life as they travel along their personal journey. It is my hope that this information will be helpful for you and your loved ones. There is power in having accurate information. I want you to feel empowered so that you can as actively and confidently as possible participate in the decision making about your treatment choices today and future treatment options that lie ahead. And know that research efforts are ongoing on your behalf, more so than ever before, to create even more treatment options, no matter what type of pathology features your metastatic breast cancer has.

Sit down, get a beverage and a soft blanket, and begin reading—and know that I am also one of the professionals cheering you on when you get good news and holding your hand from a distance when the news is bad.

A saying that is often attributed to Eleanor Roosevelt offers what I believe to be an accurate summation of what women are experiencing on their journey with this disease: "Yesterday is history; tomorrow is a mystery; today is a gift—that's why it's called 'the present.'"

Lillie Shockney, RN, BS, MAS, HON-ONN-CG

University Distinguished Service Professor of Breast Cancer

Professor of Surgery

Johns Hopkins University School of Medicine

28-year breast cancer survivor

PART ONE

Suspicions of Metastatic Breast Cancer

How is it possible for my breast cancer to come back after I did all of the treatment and my oncologist and I believed I was cancer free?

How will my oncologist decide how to treat my metastatic breast cancer?

I want to get treatment underway immediately, but everything is taking too long. Why can't I start treatment now?

More . . .

Cancer

The presence of malignant cells.

Chemotherapy

Treatment with drugs that kill cancer cells or make them less active. It is a form of systemic treatment.

Radiation therapy

The use of high-energy X-rays to kill cancer cells and shrink tumors.

Hormonal therapy

Treatment that blocks the effects of hormones on cancers.

Targeted biologic therapy

Cancer treatments that target specific characteristics of cancer cells, such as a protein, an enzyme, or the formation of new blood vessels. Targeted therapies don't harm normal healthy cells.

Oncologist

A cancer specialist who helps determine treatment choices.

Metastatic breast cancer

Cancer that has spread from the breast to other organ sites such as the liver, lung, bone, or brain.

There is a very good possibility that you have already been told that you have breast **cancer** and have undergone treatment for it. You may have had surgery, **chemotherapy**, **radiation therapy**, and maybe **hormonal therapy** or **targeted biologic therapy**. You may have come to the **oncologist's** office with complaints of back pain that you've been experiencing for the past 3 weeks that won't subside with over-the-counter pain relievers. Maybe you have headaches or some new symptom related to your breathing. Your symptoms may have triggered the doctor to order additional tests to determine if these symptoms are related to your original breast cancer diagnosis, and now you are being told that there is a chance that your new symptoms are related to **metastatic breast cancer**.

If you've been told that you might have metastatic breast cancer, it's serious for you. Every imaginable fear may be rushing through your mind. You are not alone in feeling frightened about this news. Recurrence of breast cancer is the biggest fear for all breast cancer survivors.

Though the risk of distant recurrence is higher for women with **locally advanced disease** (stage III) than with stage I or stage II disease, metastatic breast cancer can occur at any point in time after an original diagnosis of invasive breast cancer. Only women who had stage 0 or noninvasive breast cancer are considered to have no risk for metastatic breast cancer. Once you've been diagnosed with metastatic breast cancer, statistics about your risk level don't have the same meaning. Having a small risk of developing metastatic disease doesn't change the current situation.

Remember, many people can live for years with metastatic breast cancer. The cancer can be "active" sometimes and then go into **remission**. Let's walk through information about metastatic breast cancer together so that you are well informed and can participate in the decision making about your treatment and care.

1. What is metastatic breast cancer?

Breast cancer is referred to as **recurrent breast cancer** if it reappears after it was originally diagnosed and treated. Recurrence happens in two forms: **Local recurrence** means that it came back in the breast where it originally started, whereas **distant recurrence** or metastatic breast cancer means the cancer has now appeared within another part of the body, including distant organs such as the lungs, liver, bones, or brain. It is also known as stage IV breast cancer.

The goal for treatment is control of the disease while preserving your quality of life. Think of it as a chronic illness, like diabetes. If diabetics don't manage their disease by watching their diet and taking medications or insulin routinely, they will develop serious complications, like blindness or kidney failure, that affect their quality of life, and eventually they will die. Metastatic breast cancer is similar: You manage it by taking treatments regularly to keep the disease in control and, whenever possible, put it into remission so that it is not actively growing. At minimum, the goal is to maintain good quality of life for you while also treating the disease so that it remains stable over time and doesn't progress. The goal is not cure but control.

There are some situations in which a patient is diagnosed with metastatic breast cancer at the time of their initial diagnosis. This is less common, however. Most

Locally advanced disease

Stage III breast cancer.

Remission

A decrease in or disappearance of signs and symptoms of cancer.

Recurrent breast cancer

The disease has come back in spite of the initial treatment.

Local recurrence

The breast cancer has returned inside the breast after treatment was completed.

Distant recurrence

The breast cancer has been found now in another organ, such as the lungs, liver, bones, or brain. It is located outside of the breast and lymph nodes near the breast.

occur in the form of a distant recurrence some time after the patient's initial diagnosis and treatment. When breast cancer attacks other organs in the body, these organs can have difficulty doing their daily job—creating new blood **cells**, providing oxygen, metabolizing medicines, keeping our heart and lungs functioning properly, and other important processes required to sustain life.

Cell

The basic element of tissues; the appearance and composition of individual cells are unique to the tissue they compose.

2. How is it possible for my breast cancer to come back after I completed all of the treatments I was advised to do?

The treatments you received were intended to kill any breast cancer cells that remained but couldn't be seen on any scans or through other methods. Treatments don't always work 100% of the time, however; the fact that you have metastatic breast cancer means that a few breast cancer cells had already left the breast and traveled to other organ sites (such as the bones, lungs, liver, or brain) and stayed dormant. Then over some period of time, something caused those cells to start growing, multiplying, and dividing. Once the mass of cells reaches a certain size, it can cause physical symptoms that trigger your doctor to do some scans and blood work and see if the symptoms are being caused by the development of metastatic breast cancer.

Katie's comments:

I was in shock when I first heard that my cancer had returned and was in my bones. I'd had a few aches and pains that lingered longer than usual, but I never expected to hear this kind of news. The tumors in my bones are estrogen receptor-positive and HER2–positive, so the doctor said biologic targeted therapies along with hormonal therapy may get this back into control. My mission is still to live a long life with my family, and I will continue to set goals for the future.

3. I have heard that breast cancer grows more slowly in older women and doesn't need to be treated. Is that true?

Cancer is a disease of aging, and the **incidence** of breast cancer is increasing faster in older women than in younger women. As women age, their risk of breast cancer increases. Older adults with cancer often have other chronic health problems and may be taking multiple medications, both of which can affect their cancer treatment plan. Misconceptions and prejudice often prevent older patients from getting the cancer treatment that they need.

The biology of breast cancer is usually different in older women than younger women. As patients age, their breast **tumors** more frequently express **hormone receptors** (estrogen, progesterone), they have lower rates of tumor cell growth, and they're less likely to have **HER2 overexpression** (HER2 stands for *human epidermal growth factor receptor 2*). Though these are usually thought of as favorable factors, most studies show no major age-related differences in breast cancer survival. In fact, older women with **metastases** often have more aggressive disease than their younger counterparts.

Chronological age alone should not be the only factor used to determine how and when to use life-prolonging or **palliative** anticancer treatment. Despite advanced age, men and women who are relatively well often have a life expectancy that may exceed their life expectancy

Incidence
The number of times a disease occurs within a population of people.

Tumor
A mass or lump of extra tissue.

Hormone receptor
A protein on the surface or inside a cell that connects to a certain hormone (estrogen or progesterone) and causes changes in the cell.

HER2 overexpression
An excess of a certain protein (human epidermal growth factor receptor 2) on the surface of a cell that may be related to a high number of abnormal or defective cells.

Metastases, metastasize
The spread of cancer from one part of the body to another.

Palliative care
Care to relieve the symptoms of cancer and to keep the best quality of life for as long as possible.

Cancer is a disease of aging, and the incidence of breast cancer is increasing faster in older women than in younger women.

Estrogen or progesterone receptor-positive breast cancer

Cancer that uses female hormones as a fuel to grow.

Adjunct

A treatment that complements another treatment.

with breast cancer. The average 70-year-old woman is likely to live another 16 years. A similar 85-year-old can expect to live an additional six years and remain functionally independent for most of that time. Even an unwell 75-year-old probably will live five more years—long enough to experience symptoms and early death from metastatic breast cancer.

Since most older women have **estrogen** or **progesterone receptor-positive breast cancer**, commonly these patients will be placed on therapies designed for hormone receptor-positive disease. Hormonal therapy and other treatments are often an excellent treatment option. There are new **adjunct** drugs for metastatic hormone receptor-positive breast cancer patients called CDK4/6 inhibitors that make it possible to live longer and preserve quality of life, too.

It is important to mention that the health of an elderly patient, though a factor for planning her treatment, isn't as important as her overall health and well-being. Someone in a nursing home with diabetes, heart disease, and advanced dementia may die sooner from one of these illnesses than she would from breast cancer. So decisions about cancer treatment require a careful balance. Physicians must always remember the Hippocratic Oath they took—do no harm. Treatment for treatment's sake is bad care. So managing the cancer with hormonal therapy to keep it in control is likely a direction the treatment team will go.

There also are women younger than those who are considered elderly who have severe illnesses and disabilities that would impact doing aggressive treatment. What is best for each patient, based on her anticipated longevity, her symptoms (pain control is paramount), and her other medical conditions must factor into planning breast cancer care.

If the patient is older, it is beneficial to have an oncologist who specializes in the care of the elderly when the patient is much older and has other chronic illnesses that will impact treatment options.

4. How will my oncologist decide how to treat my metastatic breast cancer?

Treatment of metastatic breast cancer can prolong life and preserve quality of life, but there is no cure. Therefore, your oncologist's strategy is to get as much mileage out of each treatment regimen as possible. Since treatments with the fewest side effects are preferred, your oncologist will try to use other therapies instead of chemotherapy, whenever reasonable.

The first step in determining what possible treatment options are best for you involves looking closely at the biology of the tumor itself. This requires doing a biopsy of one of the metastatic lesions (tumors) that have grown in another organ site such as the bone, lung, liver, or brain. (For those patients with invasive lobular carcinoma, a less common form of breast cancer than invasive ductal carcinoma, the locations of the metastatic lesions might be in the stomach, uterus, ovaries, lungs, colon, and abdominal cavity.) It is very important to not merely rely on the biology of the original breast cancer in the breast or in the lymph nodes that were removed at the time of your surgery. This is because the biology of the breast cancer cells has the ability to change once it travels elsewhere. You want your metastatic breast cancer treated based on accurate information learned from the biology of the disease now found elsewhere in your body.

The assessment will include looking at the tumor cell's estrogen receptor (ER) status, the progesterone receptor (PR) status, and the HER2 receptor (HER2) status, along with the grade of the cells (which tells how fast they are growing), and other genetic factors found within the cancer cells. You will be advised to get genetically tested for breast cancer (BRCA) gene mutations, too, because there are specific treatments that are designed for patients who carry such mutations.

All of the terminology associated with the biology of the cancer cells can be confusing, so let's take a moment to explain it. "Hormone receptor-positive" means that the cancer cells have hormone receptors—structures that allow estrogen and/or progesterone to attach to a tumor cell and stimulate the cells to grow. If the tumors are estrogen receptor-positive (ER+) and/or progesterone receptor-positive (PR+), then you will likely benefit from therapies designed to block the hormones in your body from reaching the receptors on these cancer cells, which "starves" the cancer cells of the hormone(s) enabling it to grow. So being ER+ or PR+ is considered a good prognostic factor, and hormonal therapies and **CDK4/6 inhibitors** are two types of therapies that may be recommended for you.

The HER2 receptor is quite different. If the tumors are HER2−positive (HER2+), it means that the cancer cells are overexpressing an **oncogene** (a mutated form of a gene that regulates normal cell growth). It used to be that if HER2 was positive, this was considered

CDK4/6 inhibitor

A class of drugs that target enzymes called CDK4 and CDK6 that are important in cell division. CDK4/6 inhibitors are designed to interrupt the growth of cancer cells.

Oncogene

A mutated form of a gene that normally regulates cell growth, which under certain conditions can cause cancer. HER2 is an oncogene of human epidermal growth factor receptor.

a poor prognostic factor, but recent advances in cancer biology have helped to develop specific treatments known as biologic targeted therapies that are designed to get overexpression of the oncogene under control. There are also specific treatments available for those individuals who have both hormone receptor-positive and HER2+ disease, as well as special treatments for those who have hormone receptor-positive and HER2-negative (HER2–) cancer cells. The most challenging situations are those patients who have what is known as "triple negative" disease, which means that the ER, PR, and HER2 receptors are all negative—so hormone therapies and HER2 targeted therapies are ineffective, which limits the types of treatment options available.

There is also a special treatment option known as **PARP inhibitors** for patients who carry a breast cancer gene mutation. PARP is shorthand for poly (ADP-ribose) polymerase, an enzyme that helps repair damaged DNA; PARP inhibitors act by preventing PARP from helping cancer cells repair the damage done by anticancer drugs. Olaparib (*Lynparza*) is an example of a PARP inhibitor used to treat breast cancer. These drugs are used as **adjuvant therapy** to help chemotherapy work better.

PARP inhibitor

A class of drugs that blocks an enzyme involved in tumor DNA repair (called PARP enzyme). These drugs can help chemotherapy better kill cancer cells.

Right now, more research is taking place specifically in the area of metastatic breast cancer to create more feasible options to add to this war chest of treatments available today. Several exist now and are being used successfully. Though usually reserved for later in the treatment journey, **cytotoxic** chemotherapy is usually highly effective in killing breast cancer cells, too. The chemotherapy drugs you may have had before likely will not be used again; instead, other chemotherapy agents

Adjuvant therapy

Treatment given after the primary treatment to increase the chances of a cure.

Cytotoxic

A term used to describe anything that kills cells.

First-line therapy

The first drug or set of drugs that you receive as your treatment.

National Comprehensive Cancer Network (NCCN)

An organization composed of specific cancer centers across the country that excel in cancer diagnosis and treatment that work together to create treatment guidelines followed no matter where a patient is receiving care.

The order in which they choose to use these palliative agents will depend on your overall health, the organs in the body where the cancer cells have metastasized, and your track record with previous treatment regimens.

you have not received yet would probably be considered when needed.

The first drug therapy regimens given are referred to as **first-line therapy**. The next treatment after this therapy no longer is working well is called second-line therapy, and so on. Oncologists should be following evidence-based treatment guidelines that are published in peer-reviewed journals as well as published by the **National Comprehensive Cancer Network (NCCN)**. You can review these treatment guidelines yourself by visiting www.nccn.com.

5. My doctor waited for me to have symptoms before doing any scans. Could he have found my cancer earlier if he had done regular scans after my first diagnosis?

There are tests, such as **scans**, that might detect the presence of breast cancer in other organs before symptoms appear. Research studies have confirmed that doing these tests does not improve the response to treatments used and therefore doesn't translate into prolonging someone's life.

While that probably sounds strange, studies have shown it to be true. An additional issue is that performing routine scans and blood work can result in finding things that frighten the patient, only to learn after careful investigation the findings are normal and not cancer-related. Scans cannot see microscopic disease that is starting to establish itself in another organ, either. Even a scan that shows no evidence of disease isn't really a guarantee that there aren't microscopic cells growing elsewhere that can't be detected at that time.

Your doctor will focus on the areas where you have symptoms. Shortness of breath would trigger a lung scan and chest X-ray; back pain would result in a **bone scan**, for example. A blood test called CA27/29 will likely be done, as well as some routine blood chemistries to provide additional information to assist the doctors in determining the underlying cause of your symptoms. A **biopsy** is required from at least one of the organ sites where the scans are showing the potential presence of breast cancer. Your doctor might order a bone, liver, lung, or brain biopsy. Having a **pathologist** look at actual tissue from the organ provides a definitive diagnosis while enabling the oncology team to learn more about the cancer that has spread.

When you were initially diagnosed, the cancer cells in your breast were tested for specific prognostic factors. These included hormone receptors, HER2 receptors, grade of the cells, size of the tumor, **Ki67** to measure the proliferation rate of the cells, and other measurements. The tissue biopsied from the organ site also is tested in a similar way. We used to assume that the cells that traveled from the breast to distant sites would have the exact same prognostic factors as they originally had. We have learned from laboratory research that this may not be the case. When the cancer has traveled and spread, it might have converted from being hormone receptor-positive to hormone receptor-negative, for example. This information is critical to planning the right treatment options. The medicines and therapies prescribed are customized to work best on the specific cancer cells that have traveled out of your breast and are growing elsewhere in your body.

Scan

A technique to create images of specific parts of the body on a computer screen or on film.

Bone scan

An X-ray that looks for signs of metastasis to the bones.

Biopsy

A procedure in which cells are collected for microscopic examination.

Pathologist

A specialist trained to distinguish normal from abnormal cells.

Ki67

A molecule that can be easily detected in growing cells in order to gain an understanding of the rate at which the cells within a tumor are growing.

11

6. How long is it going to take before I know if I have metastatic breast cancer?

It may be challenging and frustrating for both you and your doctors to know that it can take a few days, or even a couple of weeks, to determine if you do, in fact, have metastatic breast cancer. As anxiety-provoking as that may seem, it's important that tests are done accurately, correlated with other findings, and in some cases, confirmed with biopsies done to make the diagnosis definitive before any treatment can be planned. This time frame, though it may seem prolonged to you, is important to make sure that the right things are done in the right way. Waiting a few more weeks will not alter your **prognosis** or treatment. The mission is control of the disease once it's confirmed. Knowing the pathology information and findings from scans and other X-rays is important in selecting the optimal treatment plan for you.

Prognosis

An estimation of the likely outcome of an illness based upon the patient's current status and the available treatments.

7. How did this happen? Should I have had more treatment originally when I was diagnosed?

This is a common question. Some women feel guilty; others are angry. All are certainly in shock. If you decided against a treatment you were advised to have, don't second-guess yourself. Hindsight is always 20/20. Stay focused and move forward. The question to ask yourself is, "What do I need to do *now* to get control over this disease and live in harmony with it?" If you are feeling angry, that is okay. You may feel that you have paid your dues to this disease and just found out you need to do it again, only perhaps in a scarier way. It's okay to grieve about it or be mad about it, as long as you keep moving forward with your doctors and nurses and plan your treatment. Try not to remain in an angry state, however, because you are taxing your immune system, which needs to be working well for you right now. Again, don't look backward.

Don't get on the internet, either, to try to learn all about metastatic breast cancer on your own. Online resources, even the good ones (and many aren't good), are not set up to explain *your* situation; your healthcare team is. Rely on your doctors, nurse navigator, and other professionals on your team to educate you about the *specific* type of metastatic disease you are dealing with and how to best treat it, taking your particular health factors into account.

8. I want to get treatment under way immediately, but everything is taking too long. Why can't I start treatment now?

It is in your best interest that all the test results and clinical findings are clearly understood and known before beginning treatment. There may be several different treatment options too for you to consider. You shouldn't feel rushed in making these very important decisions. Have thoughtful discussions with your oncology team. Each new doctor you see and talk to may give you new information. Remember, when you are scared and anxious, you may not process information very clearly. It can be difficult to wait patiently, but planning the treatment that is in your best interest is a goal shared by your oncology team. Taking a few weeks to iron out the best strategy will help ensure that the most appropriate

decisions have been made to give you the best opportunity for living in harmony with this disease and managing it as a chronic, but serious, illness. This is the time
for thoughtful and wise decisions. So don't go running
around to different doctors to find someone who will
start quickly, because the treatment that is used first
may not be the best possible treatment—and it can prevent you from getting the right treatments in the right
order at the right time at the right dosage.

If you live in a rural area where oncologists may be few
in number, at a minimum get a second opinion at a large
comprehensive cancer center so your treatment plan is
established by breast cancer experts who care for a large
volume of patients like you with stage IV breast cancer.

PART TWO

Ensuring You Are in Good Hands—Selecting the Multidisciplinary Oncology Team to Take Care of You

How do I know I'm receiving the best and most appropriate care for my current situation?

How can I participate in the decision making about my treatment?

How do I select a medical oncologist who will be primarily responsible for my care and treatments?

More . . .

9. How do I know I'm receiving the best and most appropriate care for my current situation?

It would seem to make perfect sense to be taken care of by the oncology team who originally treated you for breast cancer. Your clinical situation is now much more serious than perhaps it was at that time. There are some steps you may want to take to ensure that this is the most appropriate team to continue managing your care.

You can't judge a breast center's quality based on the facility's advertisements. Sometimes it requires a lot of effort on your part (or someone else's, on your behalf) to do the necessary due diligence to ensure that you are in good hands. A breast center that is part of a National Cancer Institute (NCI)-designated cancer center is usually a wise choice.

There are many services and programs that a patient should be seeking from a breast center when she is initially diagnosed and treated. For women dealing with metastatic breast cancer, there are some specific features that you want to be sure are available to you. They include:

Patient empowerment. It's important that you be given the knowledge you need to enable you to actively participate in the decisions about your care and treatment. Some physicians are reluctant to empower women in this way. Make sure that your team understands that you expect this.

You can't judge a breast center's quality based on the facility's advertisements.

Patient and family education. Not only do you need to be educated—so does your family. You *and* they need to know what to expect—when, how, and why. You need easy access to someone who will be able to support you and respond to your questions as you take this critical journey. It is important to receive written literature as well as verbal information.

Multidisciplinary case conferences and tumor board meetings. The key advantage to having a multidisciplinary team approach is the special expertise each healthcare professional offers to the patient's unique situation. Centers that hold weekly breast cancer conferences can provide that. There may be times that your next steps for treatment decision making are unclear to both you and your doctor. Your doctor can present your case to the entire team in this setting and get input on your behalf. There is great value in having oncology specialists who specialize in breast cancer and see and treat a large volume of breast cancer patients, including those with stage IV breast cancer that has the same prognostic factors as your cancer does.

Access to **clinical trials.** This may be one of the most important times that you want to ensure you have access to clinical trials that may offer additional benefits to controlling this disease. These clinical trials would include all **phases** of research study.

Breast medical oncologists. You want to ensure that the medical oncologist taking care of you specializes in breast cancer and has expertise in women with metastatic disease.

Breast radiation oncologists. There may be a need for radiation during your treatment, so you want to ensure that the radiation oncologist specializes in breast cancer and has expertise in treating women with metastatic disease.

Clinical trial

Research study in which patients are offered the opportunity to try new, innovative therapies (under careful observation) in order to help doctors identify the best treatments with the fewest side effects. These studies help improve the overall standard of care.

Phase

A series of steps followed in clinical trials.

Pathology services. Patients don't always think about this particular service, but it is a very important one. The pathologist who looks at your tissue specimen determines the prognostic factors, and the rest of the team uses that information to formulate a treatment plan. Accuracy and completeness are critical.

Some say that the pathologist "holds all the cards" because his or her opinion about what is on your pathology slides is critical information. We don't want to overtreat or undertreat a patient, but this happens every day because there are no clear standards regarding pathology interpretation. A breast center that has pathologists who specialize in breast pathology has an edge since they are likely to see higher volume than other pathologists. They have also made a commitment to specialize in breast disease.

Although you have been diagnosed and know your tumor's prognostic factors, there may be times in which additional biopsies are needed. For example, you will need biopsies of other organ sites. The pathology from other organ sites where the breast cancer may have spread will be compared to the original pathology found in the breast tumor itself. Sometimes it is discovered that the prognostic factors (like hormone receptors and HER2) have changed. You want a facility that has pathologists who specialize in breast pathology because their accuracy is critical to planning your treatment. These types of accuracy and precision are very important in planning the optimal treatment for your specific pathology situation.

Breast cancer nurse navigators. There are oncology **nurse navigators** who specialize in breast cancer and even some who specialize in navigating and supporting those

Nurse navigator

A healthcare professional who assists patients in navigating their care and treatment by helping them with scheduling appointments, answering questions related to test results, and offering patient education, support, and guidance in decision-making across the continuum of care.

who have metastatic disease. This type of nurse is edu-cating and supporting you as well as serving usually as your "go-to" person on the multidisciplinary team. She attends tumor board meetings and case conferences and can serve as your voice addressing questions that may arise. She also is there to support family members. Coordination of care is her specialty too. She will iden-tify any barriers to care you may have such as transpor-tation, financial, and work issues and provide resources for overcoming them too.

Palliative care specialists. The term *palliative care* is often misunderstood. It is commonly only mentioned when someone is discussing hospice, but palliative care fo-cuses on symptom control, not end-of-life care. Think of palliative care as quality-of-life preservation or res-toration, because quality of life is what palliative care is all about. Even before you need such a specialist, it is important to learn if such a specialist is on your team and available whenever needed. They can help you manage pain, peripheral neuropathy, joint stiffness, nausea, loss of appetite, fatigue, and other symptoms. They also work hard to not use opioids as the method of solving the problem.

NCCN treatment guidelines. The care that results in the best outcomes is care that meets specific standards of quality. The NCCN treatment guidelines are the gold standard for the treatment of each type and stage of cancer. Inquire if your team is using these standards in planning your treatment.

Effective communication among the team members. There needs to be good communication among your team members, and that includes you. Find out how they go about communicating information to you as well as to one another. Most use electronic patient records, as well as email, and discussions at weekly tumor board meetings.

Shared-care model of care. All too often, the patient's **primary care provider (PCP)** no longer sees the patient once cancer has been diagnosed, and especially if metastatic disease is found. Ideally, however, your PCP should remain part of your new treatment team, continuing to manage your other illnesses and disorders, making sure your vaccines are given when due, and staying involved as needed.

Primary care provider (PCP)

The patient's normal healthcare provider, usually an internal medicine or family medicine practitioner.

Patient-centered care. The patient is far more than their pathology. You may have stage IV breast cancer, but you also are a 44-year-old woman who is divorced, raising a 9-year-old with autism, working as a fifth-grade school teacher, and loves knitting and watching college football. You need to make sure you are being treated as a person, with a life that you want to continue living while getting your treatment. The milestones that are coming up soon needs to be known to the team so they are preserved for you, such as your son's special musical happening in four weeks at his school where he has a character role. You don't want to be starting a new treatment a day or so before this important event occurs. So make sure that what's important to you is known and preserved by your team.

Urgent care needs. When an urgent problem arises, such as spiking a fever, you need to have ready access to a healthcare professional who is easy to reach and who knows how to manage your medical needs promptly. Inquire about how such issues are handled.

Breast surgical oncologist. There may be a need for surgery at some point. Some oncologists are recommending removal of the breast to rid the body of the source of the disease. There are also unfortunate situations in which the tumor should be removed for pain control.

Interventional radiologist. Sometimes there is a need for procedures that involve the skills of a radiologist who can do nerve blocks or other types of procedures for palliative care purposes or even for diagnosing whether cancer has spread further to other organs.

Cancer rehabilitation. Keeping active is important to your quality of life. Rehabilitation therapists can help with this element of your care. They can also show your family members how to preserve your energy for special events you want to attend.

Emotional support. Clearly, this is part of your treatment. Inquire what services are available for supporting you and your family. You'll want to ask about psychological support, as well as financial assistance in case issues arise and money is tight due to missing time from work.

Jill's comments:

I originally had my breast cancer treatment 2 years ago at a local hospital. Things went fine. But now that I'm dealing with metastatic disease, I really want to be sure that I am in the best of hands to provide me the optimal treatment for longevity and quality of life. So I went to an NCI-designated comprehensive cancer center. I'm being taken care of by an experienced team of doctors and nurses who deal with this kind of situation every day. That gives me great peace of mind.

Patients deserve to be empowered so that they can actively participate in decisions about their care and treatment.

10. How can I participate in the decision making about my treatment?

Patients deserve to be empowered so that they can actively participate in decisions about their care and treatment. Some physicians are reluctant to empower women in this way. It is a patient's right and should be a key factor in deciding where she wants to receive her treatment. Seek an oncology team that specializes in breast cancer and has a great deal of experience in treating and managing patients with metastatic disease. The purpose of treating your metastatic breast cancer is to help you live as long as possible with a good quality of life. Since different people have different beliefs and values, it is important that you communicate these to your healthcare team so that everyone can be working for the same goals.

Studies show that the more we empower a patient and give her a solid knowledge base about her breast cancer, the more satisfied she is with her care. This includes educating other family members when appropriate. There will be family members who will be helping with your care, so they need to understand the treatment plan and know what to expect.

11. I've heard the term **multidisciplinary care** or **tumor board** used. What are these, and should I be requesting them for myself?

A key advantage to having a multidisciplinary team approach is the special expertise each healthcare professional offers to each patient's unique situation. Centers that hold weekly breast cancer case conferences (sometimes referred to as *breast cancer tumor boards*) to discuss in detail a patient's clinical condition, diagnostic findings, and recommendations for optimal treatment find that these meetings are beneficial to the patient's overall well-being and clinical outcome. Since your case will be discussed in light of the most up-to-date research findings, this is a way that you can ensure that you are being given individualized attention and care by a team of experts. All National Cancer Institute–accredited cancer centers are required to conduct such conferences on a regular basis and maintain records of the cases presented. So are cancer centers accredited by the Commission on Cancer. Usually, the patient is informed by the physician presenting her case that her clinical situation is going to be discussed by the team. The doctor then informs the patient of the discussion and outcome of that presentation, including clinical research trials that the patient may choose to participate in. Ask your doctor if she is part of a multidisciplinary team and if your case will be presented at their tumor board meeting.

12. Why would I be participating in a clinical trial now? I thought that they were just for women with breast cancer that hasn't spread.

Having as many treatment options available to you as possible can be valuable. Breast centers that participate in clinical trials can usually offer more innovative treatment options. Many clinical trials offer you treatment that is at least as good as the **standard of care**—and possibly better. If you are asked to participate in such a trial, you are also paving the way for the development of innovative research that will make an important impact

Standard of care

A diagnostic and treatment process that a clinician should follow for a certain type of patient, illness, or clinical circumstance.

Breast centers that partici- pate in clini- cal trials can usually offer more innova- tive treatment options.

on other women diagnosed in the future. You will be closely monitored throughout the treatment process so that data can be collected about your experience with the chemotherapy agents you've been given. For more on clinical trials, see Questions 75–78 in Part Eight. There are also resources in the Appendix that can help you find clinical trials nationwide.

13. My surgery was done when I was originally diagnosed with breast cancer. Will I still need a breast surgeon to be involved now?

You probably had breast cancer surgery when you were originally diagnosed. There *are* situations, however, that result in needing additional surgery when breast can- cer returns. This can be for local control of the disease, diagnostic purposes, or to relieve pain. It is preferable that the surgeon is a **surgical oncologist** who special- izes in breast cancer. Such surgeons are often found at a large teaching hospital that is part of a comprehensive cancer center. There may also be a need for some pa- tients to have a plastic surgeon who specializes in breast reconstruction.

Surgical oncologist

A surgeon who spe- cializes in removing cancerous tumors and has had addi- tional surgical train- ing to specialize solely in operating on cancer.

14. How do I select the medical oncologist who will be primarily responsible for my care and treatments?

You will feel more confident being treated by a medi- cal oncologist who specializes in breast cancer and very experienced with treatment of stage IV breast cancer.

You will want someone who treats a large volume of women with this disease and has access to a spectrum of clinical trials for you to consider. Be sure also to ask how the physician's office practice handles emergency issues, such as a sudden high fever or uncontrolled nausea and vomiting. You will also want to know who will cover for your doctor on weekends or when he or she is on vacation. This "backup doctor" should also be a medical oncologist. These are important factors to ask about so that you are confident your case is being well managed.

Ask what education is available to help you prepare for known side effects of treatment. Inquire how patients are referred for wig fittings, as well as any skin-care needs that may occur during treatment. Some breast centers offer these services within their facility.

15. Do I need a radiation oncologist?

Most patients who have had breast conservation surgery (lumpectomy) or have had locally advanced disease have already undergone radiation therapy in some manner. It is valuable to go to a facility that has extensive experience as well as doctors and therapists who specialize in treating this specific type of cancer. They will have a **radiation physicist** on staff who assists with the treatment planning. There are different methods of delivering radiation for breast cancer treatment today. Some are part of clinical trials and some are standard of care. Patients will want to know how their heart and lungs will be protected from the radiation. At some point during your treatment for metastatic disease, you may need radiation therapy to help shrink the tumor(s), provide local

Radiation physicist

A specialist who makes sure that radiotherapy equipment is working properly and that the machines deliver the right dose of radiation.

control of the disease, or reduce pain symptoms (see Questions 23–25 for more on radiation therapy).

16. How do I make sure my medical oncologist, radiation oncologist, and family doctor are communicating with one another and not relying on me to give them updates?

You need to have confidence that you are being watched over and cared for appropriately. Most facilities have nurse practitioners and nurse navigators who stay in touch with the patients via telephone once they are home from surgery and/or chemotherapy. **Nurse navigators** help with coordination of care and eliminate any barriers you may have that would impact your getting care, such as lack of transportation or financial barriers that result in large copayments and deductibles.

The team of professionals taking care of you also needs to stay in close contact with one another. Tumor board conferences (Question 11) are another way that your team stays in touch. Ask them how they communicate and keep each other informed about your condition and needs. You want to know that you are being cared for by a team who stays well connected with you and with each other. Feeling confident that you are receiving good continuity of care provides wonderful peace of mind to you and your family. Consider your nurse navigator as your go-to person for questions. Also, most facilities use electronic patient records, which work well in communicating to you and vice versa. One example is a widely used communication tool called MyChart.

Nurse navigator

A healthcare professional who assists patients in navigating their care and treatment by helping them with scheduling appointments, answering questions related to test results, and offering patient education, support, and guidance in decision making across the continuum of care.

You want to know that you are being cared for by a team who stays well connected with you and with each other.

17. Who do I call when I have an emergency or urgent problem?

When an urgent medical problem arises, such as vomiting that won't subside, a clear process needs to be in place for patient management. Ask what the doctor's procedures are for handling such emergencies. A breast center needs to have available a professional healthcare provider 24 hours a day, 7 days a week to handle emergencies. In addition to this, patients should know how to access this service and know they can confidently rely on it. Though it is hoped that you will not need such services, it's important they are in place and can be readily accessed.

18. The stress of thinking about what may lie ahead is overwhelming to me. Who can help me with these feelings?

You need to be treated as a total person. You are not only a stage IV breast cancer patient. You may be a school teacher, recently divorced, with two young children who has a mother with chronic illnesses who lives with you. Breast centers usually provide social work counseling, psychotherapy services, nurse navigators, and nurses along with others to help you along this journey. Some offer to match a breast cancer patient with a survivor volunteer based on her age, stage of disease, and anticipated treatment plan, including those with metastatic disease. This isn't always possible, but when it is, it provides a unique level of support for someone just embarking on chronic treatment. Patients usually value the opportunity to talk with others. Some breast centers also offer special support groups for women dealing with metastatic disease.

Breast centers like Johns Hopkins offer special retreats for women with stage IV breast cancer. These events are designed to help patients and their family members as they take the journey together as a family with the treatment of this disease. Such programs, funded by generous donors, can help a patient make decisions regarding continuation of treatment, define quality of life from her perspective, and ensure that her voice is heard when it comes to treatment and end-of-life wishes. There programs are not limited to Johns Hopkins patients, so for more information, email me (Lillie Shockney) at shockli@jhmi.edu.

I am also assisting other breast cancer centers nationally in orchestrating the same type of retreat. Many of these types of retreats are funded by philanthropy or foundations such as the National Breast Cancer Foundation. There are also annual conferences held by Living Beyond Breast Cancer; Susan G. Komen; and Theresa's Foundation. Watch for these educational programs as well and plan to attend if you want to learn more about research endeavors associated with this disease and its treatment as well as to network with others.

PART THREE

Decisions Regarding Surgery and Radiation for the Treatment of Metastatic Breast Cancer

My cancer has spread to my brain and is located in one spot. What are the treatment options for this type of metastasis?

How is radiation used for the treatment or control of metastatic breast cancer?

I've had radiation already to shrink the cancer in my spine, and it has regrown. Can I have radiation again?

More . . .

If you've been diagnosed with and treated for breast cancer in the past, you more than likely had either a **lumpectomy** or **mastectomy**. If this is your first breast cancer diagnosis, and it was discovered from the outset that the cancer has spread to other organs, then you probably haven't had any surgery. The following is some information related to surgical decisions and what you might expect.

Lumpectomy

Breast cancer surgery to remove the breast cancer and a small amount of normal tissue surrounding it.

Mastectomy

Surgery that removes the whole breast.

19. I had a lumpectomy and axillary node dissection done three years ago, and now the cancer has returned to my bones. Will the doctor need to do a mastectomy now?

No, the concern isn't about breast cancer still being in your breast. The surgery or radiation that you had three years ago took care of that. The issue now is treating the disease that has spread elsewhere. The time has come for **systemic treatment**, which is treatment that will travel throughout your body no matter where the cancer cells may have gone. Medicines are used to treat disease when it has spread. If you are experiencing bone pain, radiation may also be given to shrink a specific area where a tumor exists that is pressing on nerves and causing the pain.

Systemic treatment

Treatment that targets cancer cells anywhere in the body.

Chrissie's comments:

I was really hoping that the doctor would simply tell me that I can have a mastectomy and some pills to treat my cancer. Having now met with her and understanding my situation better, I realize that doing surgery isn't the first priority; treating the disease where it has spread needs to be my first focus.

20. My cancer has spread to my brain and is located in one spot. What are the treatment options for this type of metastasis?

Sometimes when the cancer is in one specific spot and is relatively small, it can be surgically treated, including when it is found in the brain. A neurosurgeon would be consulted about this type of surgical procedure. More than likely, this type of surgery would be followed by radiation to the brain. There are also other times that radiation alone is used to shrink cancer that has metastasized to the brain.

Andrea's comments:

Learning my cancer had spread to my brain was devastating. I had been having headaches, something that rarely happens to me. The cancer is in one spot, and the doctors said that it could probably be surgically removed. This gives me great hope for the future that I'll be around longer to spend time with my children.

Sometimes when the cancer is in one specific spot and is relatively small, it can be surgically treated, including when it is found to be in the brain.

21. I have disease in my liver. Can I get a liver transplant as my treatment?

Unfortunately, no. Liver transplants are more for treatment of disease in the liver that is not cancer-related. Liver transplants are not often used for metastatic disease because there is a high incidence of undetectable micrometastases elsewhere and recurrence is highly likely.

When the cancer in the liver is limited to just one small area, it can sometimes be removed using techniques called **ablation** that can destroy cancer cells in one

Ablation

A nonsurgical technique for destroying cancerous tissue using heat or cold delivered directly to the tumor site.

small area using special instruments. Ablation eliminates tumors without surgery using one of several forms of energy to select which tumors to ablate. This procedure can be done with minimally invasive techniques on an outpatient basis (no hospital stay needed).

Radiofrequency ablation

A tumor ablation method that relies on radio waves to create heat energy to destroy cancer cells.

Microwave ablation

A tumor ablation method that relies on microwaves to create heat energy to destroy cancer cells.

Cryoablation

A tumor ablation method that delivers cold gas to a tumor in order to kill cancer cells by freezing them.

Radiologists can deliver tumor-eliminating energy through a needlelike probe that they insert through the skin and guide into the tumor with the help of advanced imaging technologies.

The most common ablation methods destroy the cancerous tissue through the application of heat delivered by radio waves (**radiofrequency ablation**) or microwaves (**microwave ablation**) or through cold gas that freezes the tumor (**cryoablation**).

Ablation is most often used when there is just a single metastatic breast cancer tumor within the liver. When there are several tumors or one large tumor, usually this technique is not recommended, and systemic treatments that treat the entire body, including the liver, are used instead. These systemic treatments usually involve medications.

22. I haven't had surgery of any kind yet because when my cancer was discovered, it was found to have already spread to my bones. Based on my scans, the cancer is now in control. Will the doctor consider doing breast cancer surgery and radiation now?

When breast cancer is in control or only small amounts of disease have been found in another organ site, more and more women are having breast cancer surgery. The size of the original tumor in the breast determines if a lumpectomy or mastectomy would be most appropriate. This rids the body of the source of the disease, and some studies have shown that, when it is possible to do this type of procedure, it may prolong survival. The clinical circumstances have to be very specific, however, so not everyone is a candidate.

23. How is radiation used for the treatment or control of metastatic breast cancer?

Radiation is considered local treatment and is designed to treat cancerous tissue in a specific, well-defined area. Women who have had a lumpectomy for the treatment of their original breast cancer more than likely had radiation of the breast following that surgery to prevent local recurrence of the breast cancer. But when you have metastatic breast cancer—either as your initial diagnosis or as a recurrence—you are dealing with a different situation. The breast cancer has spread (or returned) to a distant organ outside of the breast where it first began. At this point, cancer cells could be anywhere in your body—and irradiating your whole body is not a realistic option. So systemic treatments using medications (Question 27) are the cornerstone of your treatment now.

Even in metastatic breast cancer, however, radiation can be used in a variety of ways. It can be used to shrink the tumors, to control pain caused by the tumors, and, for small tumors, to directly treat the tumor until it disappears. Cancers that have spread to the bone are sometimes treated this way if they are causing pain and/or are limited to just a few specific spots. Radiation is also used to treat and control brain metastases.

Emily's comments:

The pain I was having in my back was unbearable for a while until the doctor decided to do radiation. I would never have imagined that doing a couple weeks of daily radiation would have taken nearly all of my back pain away, but it did. What a relief to feel more like myself and regain my quality of life.

24. How does the doctor protect the rest of my body from getting radiation it doesn't need?

With the help of 3D imaging, computed tomography (CT) scans, magnetic resonance imaging (MRI), and a physicist, the radiation oncology team can plan your radiation therapy so that it targets the specific areas that need treatment. "Blocks" are also created to help protect other vital organs and tissue from receiving radiation. Some tissue may be irradiated that is at the edge of the radiation field. The doctor will discuss with you what side effects you may experience, if any, and how long they will last. (See Part 6 for information on side effects.) Radiation in general is well tolerated, with the primary side effect being fatigue.

25. I've had radiation already to shrink the cancer in my spine, but it has regrown. Can I have radiation again?

Your radiation oncologist needs to carefully review the amount of radiation you have received thus far to determine if you can have more in that specific area of the spine. There is a maximum recommended dosage that one should not exceed. Records are kept of the dosages you received for each treatment so that this can be tracked and factored into the decision making about further radiation if and when it is needed.

PART FOUR

Systemic Therapy for the Treatment of Metastatic Disease

What does systemic treatment versus local treatment mean?

What are the various categories of systemic treatment, and how do they work?

I got really strong chemotherapy treatments that included several drugs when I was originally diagnosed. Why am I only getting a pill now?

How will the doctor determine if the treatments I am receiving are actually working?

More . . .

26. What does systemic treatment versus local treatment mean?

Systemic treatment consists of drugs that treat the entire body, so wherever the cancer cells might be, these drugs find and kill them. Local treatment is designed to kill or remove cancer cells found in a specific area of the body. If you had treatment for an earlier-stage breast cancer in the past, then you likely had local treatment in the form of breast cancer surgery (lumpectomy or mastectomy with or without lymph nodes removed) and possibly also radiation therapy. These two procedures only focused on the specific place where the cancer started and where it potentially traveled to, that being the lymph nodes under your arm. The surgery was intended to remove the original tumor as well as a margin of tissue around the tumor to help make sure all of the cancer is gone from the breast area. The radiation was given to eradicate any lingering cancer cells that still might be hidden in the breast. The radiation also might have been used in your underarm and chest wall area, particularly if lymph nodes containing cancer were found when the surgery was performed. You may have had additional treatments in the form of systemic treatment back then, too. When you got adjuvant chemotherapy, the hope was that it would eradicate all of the **micrometastases** that were in your body. Unfortunately, that did not work, and those cells have now grown into obvious metastases.

Micrometastasis

A small number of cancer cells that have spread from the primary tumor to other parts of the body and are too few to be picked up in a screening or diagnostic test.

It does not make any sense to treat your cancer with drugs to which it is already resistant. Therefore, your oncologist will probably want to choose new drugs to fight your cancer. This is especially true if your cancer returned while you were getting those drugs or shortly after you stopped taking them.

27. What are the various forms of systemic therapy, and how do they work?

The main forms of systemic therapy are chemotherapy, hormonal therapy, biologic targeted therapy, immunotherapy, PARP inhibitors, and CDK4/6 inhibitors. Chemotherapy and hormonal therapy have been around for many years. Biologic targeted therapies and immunotherapy are newer but have proven very beneficial in specific situations. PARP and CDK4/6 inhibitors are the newest of all and represent an exciting development in cancer treatment. We'll look at each in turn.

Chemotherapy

Chemotherapy ("chemo") is a cancer treatment that uses medicines to stop the growth of cancer cells. Technically, drugs that kill bacteria and other germs are also called chemotherapy, but the term is most commonly used to refer to cancer-killing drugs. This type of treatment has been around for many decades. New forms of chemotherapy are being developed all the time, along with newer systemic therapy **agents**.

Agent

A specific medication that can be used alone or in combination with another agent to treat cancer.

Although most people think of chemotherapy as intravenous infusions, it can also be taken by mouth or injected into a muscle. Because the chemotherapy eventually gets into the bloodstream, all three of these methods of administration allow the chemotherapy to attack cancer cells at sites great distances from the original cancer. Sometimes it is better to place the chemotherapy directly into an organ like the liver, into the spinal fluid, or into a body cavity like the peritoneum (abdominal cavity) or pleura (chest cavity). This

Chemotherapy ("chemo") is a cancer treatment that uses medicines to stop the growth of cancer cells.

is usually done in conjunction with the body-wide (systemic) treatment, but not always.

Chemotherapy drugs work in a variety of ways, but they all work by killing cancer cells or stopping them from growing. However, most chemotherapy drugs are not too smart. These cytotoxic drugs work by killing fast-growing cells, but they cannot tell the difference between a cancer cell and a healthy cell. Cancer cells grow much faster than even the fastest-growing normal cells. If the cell is unable to reproduce, it will eventually die without another cell to replace it. This results in a decrease in the number of cancer cells. Some normal cells grow very slowly, and others, like hair, blood cells, and the cells lining the gastrointestinal tract, grow relatively fast. That is why side effects of chemotherapy may include low blood cell counts, mouth sores, diarrhea, hair loss, and infertility.

Jessica's comments:

Losing my hair again was devastating to me. I was so excited before when it grew back after my chemo. Now it's gone again, and I don't know if it will grow back based on all the medicines I'm taking. That may seem like a petty issue to most people, but for me, seeing my own hair back on my head meant that I was healthy again. So seeing that it is gone and having others know it is gone represents illness that I find very scary. It would be easier for me if the treatments I had didn't cause hair loss. The doctors feel that chemotherapy, however, is my best option right now, so I'll do what I have to do to keep fighting off this disease.

Hormonal Therapy

First, let's discuss what hormones are. **Hormones** are biochemicals that send "messages" to the body's cells and tissues, affecting how these cells and tissues behave. They are produced in various locations in the body and often travel through the bloodstream to reach their target tissues. They pass on their "messages" by binding to proteins in the cell's membrane called **hormone receptors**. These proteins become activated when the specific hormone binds to them, and their activity causes a change in the cell's behavior.

Consider the sex hormones **estrogen** and **progesterone** as two examples relevant to breast cancer. These hormones are produced by the ovaries in women during their reproductive years (after puberty but before menopause) and are also produced by some other tissues, including the adrenal glands, fat, and skin. We tend to think of them as "female sex hormones" because they are so crucial in the development and maintenance of female sex characteristics and the menstrual cycle and pregnancy, but they have other roles to play in men as well as in women—for both sexes, estrogen is important for the growth and maintenance of strong bones, and progesterone has important effects on the brain and nervous system.

Some breast cancer cells have receptors for estrogen, progesterone, or both. When activated, these receptors cause specific genes to "turn on" or "turn off," which can stimulate the cancerous cell's growth or suppress the normal processes that would cause the cell's death. Either (or both) of these changes allow the cell to grow and reproduce into a tumor. Such

Hormone
Chemical messengers in the body.

Estrogen
Female hormone related to child bearing.

Progesterone
A steroid hormone belonging to a class of hormones called progestogens.

cancers are called **hormone-sensitive** (or hormone-dependent) breast cancers, because their interaction with estrogen, progesterone, or both is what produces their growth.

It makes sense that if a hormone produces these effects in cancer cells, the best way to treat hormone-dependent cancers is to stop them from interacting with that hormone. This is the goal of hormonal therapy (also called endocrine therapy): It either blocks the body's ability to produce specific hormones (so there are no hormones to help cancer cells grow) or it interferes with the effects of hormones on breast cancer cells by preventing the hormone from binding to its receptor.

To determine whether breast cancer cells contain estrogen and/or progesterone receptors, doctors test samples of tumor tissue that have been removed by a biopsy or surgery. If the tumor cells contain estrogen receptors, the cancer is estrogen receptor-positive (ER+), which means it responds to estrogen. Similarly, if the tumor cells contain progesterone receptors, the cancer is progesterone receptor-positive (PR+) and responds to progesterone. A great majority (80%) of breast cancers are ER+, and many ER+ breast cancers are also PR+. If a tumor lacks a receptor for either estrogen or progesterone, it is considered estrogen or progesterone receptor-negative (ER– or PR–). It's important to specify when a receptor is *not* present so treatment will focus on blocking only the receptors that *are* present in the cancer. There are some breast cancers that have neither estrogen nor progesterone receptors. These are sometimes called hormone receptor-negative (HR–). The details of hormonal therapy are described in Questions 39–44.

As an aside, breast cancers that are hormone sensitive are sometimes referred to as hormone receptor-positive or HR-positive. It's important not to confuse this with HER2+; HER2 is not a hormone, and HER2+ breast cancer is a completely different consideration that we'll discuss in brief below and in detail in Questions 45–54.

Hormonal therapy for breast cancer also should not be confused with the hormonal treatment used to help relieve symptoms of menopause, which was formerly called hormone replacement therapy (HRT) and is now commonly called *menopause hormone therapy* (MHT). MHT is intended to stimulate hormone receptors in normal tissues, whereas hormonal therapy for breast cancer blocks hormone receptors to prevent tumor growth. MHT can stimulate the growth of ER+ or PR+ breast cancer cells, which is why a woman diagnosed with a hormone-sensitive breast cancer is instructed to stop using MHT.

Biologic Targeted Therapy

In recent years, clinical trials have been conducted to evaluate the effectiveness of new drugs that alter the behavior of the breast cancer cell. These drugs are referred to as *biologic targeted therapy*, or sometimes just "targeted therapy" or "biologics." Biologic targeted therapies are developed specifically to attack a particular aspect of the cancer cell's biology with the goal of either stopping its growth or encouraging it to die.

One example of targeted therapy for breast cancer is directed at a gene called human epidermal growth receptor 2 (HER2) that helps control how cells grow, divide, and repair themselves. The HER2 gene directs the production of a special receptor that helps breast cells grow normally. However, if there are too many copies of the gene within the cell, or if the gene produces too many of its receptors (what's called **HER2 overexpression**), the breast cells then have the ability to turn into a breast cancer cell. These breast cancers are called HER2+. Overexpressed HER2 receptors are found in about 20 to 25% of breast cancers, and such cancers are considered particularly aggressive.

HER2 overexpression

An excess of a certain protein (HER2) on the surface of a cell that may be related to a high number of abnormal or defective cells.

Biologic targeted therapies are available that zero in specifically on the HER2 receptor; these are used to stop the growth of HER2+ breast cancer cells. HER2–targeted therapy may be given with chemotherapy to shrink a breast cancer before surgery or to prevent the cancer from coming back after surgery. HER2–targeted therapy also can be used to control a breast cancer that has spread to other parts of the body. However, if your breast cancer is not HER2+, you will not benefit from HER2–targeted therapy.

Special tests such as immunohistochemistry (IHC) or fluorescence in situ hybridization (FISH) are used by the pathologist to determine if the breast cancer cells are HER2+ or HER2–. If they're positive, a patient may be advised to take targeted biologic therapy. Treatment of HER2+ cancer is discussed in detail in Part 6 (Questions 45–54).

PARP Inhibitors

Systemic treatments are getting more and more sophisticated and are truly functioning as therapies that have the ability to biologically and physiologically work within the breast cancer cells themselves to stop their continued growth and survival within the body. PARP inhibitors are a good example of this type of innovative treatment.

The poly (ADP-ribose) polymerase (PARP) enzyme fixes DNA damage in both healthy and cancerous cells. Research has shown that medicines that interfere with or inhibit the PARP enzyme make it even harder for cancer cells with breast cancer–related gene mutations called *BRCA1* and *BRCA2* to fix DNA damage done by radiation or chemotherapy. In other words, a PARP inhibitor makes some cancer cells less likely to survive treatment. PARP inhibitors such as olaparib (*Lynparza*) and talazoparib (*Talzenna*) have been approved to treat advanced-stage HER2– breast cancer in people with a *BRCA1* or *BRCA2* mutation.

CDK4/6 Inhibitors

Another relatively new and innovative treatment is CDK4/6 inhibitor therapy, which is a targeted treatment that works within the breast cancer cell itself. CDK4/6 inhibitors are a class of drugs that target enzymes important in cell division called CDK4 and CDK6. By suppressing these key enzymes, CDK4/6 inhibitors are designed to interrupt the growth of cancer cells. These drugs are used in combination with hormone therapy to treat hormone receptor-positive, HER2– metastatic breast cancers. The CDK4/6 inhibitors currently used to treat metastatic breast cancer are abemaciclib (*Verzenio*), palbociclib (*Ibrance*), and ribociclib (*Kisqali*). Abemaciclib may also be used alone to treat these cancers.

Immunotherapy

Immunotherapy medicines work by helping your immune system work harder or smarter to attack cancer cells. Atezolizumab (*Tecentriq*) is an immune checkpoint inhibitor, which means it targets a specific protein that helps cancer cells hide from the immune system—in this case, the PD-L1 protein. By inhibiting PD-L1, the drug essentially allows immune system cells to "see" the cancer cells and kill them.

The immune checkpoint inhibitor atezolizumab is used in combination with the chemotherapy medicine nab-paclitaxel (*Abraxane*) as a first-line treatment for tumors that can't be removed surgically and that is locally advanced or metastatic HR– and HER2– breast cancer.

28. I got really strong chemotherapy treatments that included several drugs when I was originally diagnosed. Why am I only getting a pill now?

The mission of treatment is control of the cancer and to treat it as a chronic, but serious, disease. Don't discount the power of a pill. More and more cancer treatments are being developed specifically for oral administration so that you can have the freedom of spending your time away from the infusion center. Each therapy is given for as long as it is working for you. When it stops working, then a different therapy will be recommended and given. As each therapy stops working, usually the next treatment may have more side effects and also may not work as long as the prior therapy did. This isn't always the case, but it usually is. So the pill you are taking now is designed to work, hopefully for a long time. As you go from one therapy to another, however, the length of time that a new treatment works may be shorter. Very toxic treatments are usually reserved for much later because they are hard on your body and have probably limited benefit. There will be times that your doctor will have you on several drugs at the same time.

Chemotherapy works by killing cancer cells. There are a number of ways to do this, and different drugs attack cancer cells in different ways. If a mugger in a dark alley attacked you, you probably would not just hit him in the stomach. You would have a better chance of stopping him if you hit him in several vulnerable spots—stomach, head, back, and groin. When oncologists choose to use several anticancer drugs (**combination chemotherapy**) they are doing the biological equivalent of your multipronged attack on the mugger.

Combination chemotherapy
Treatment using more than one anticancer drug at a time.

The downside of this approach is that the combined drugs have more side effects than single drugs. Breast cancer that has not metastasized is potentially curable, and oncologists pull out all the stops to do this, even if there is a chance of more toxicity. Most people are willing to accept the short-term risk of toxicity if there is a reasonable chance that the chemotherapy will cure their cancer. Unfortunately, when breast cancer has recurred or spread, it cannot be totally eliminated, and there is a need to make big changes in how it is treated. The goal of treatment is no longer to cure the disease, it's to extend your life while also allowing you to enjoy your life for as long as possible. Depending on the **prognostic factors** of your breast cancer and how well the treatments are working, this time frame may be a few years to even decades. Since you will likely be getting some form of anticancer treatment for the rest of your life, doctors

Prognostic factors
Identifiable features of the cancer that help determine how best to treat it and what its long-term prognosis may be.

need to balance your quality of life with the side effects that the treatment will cause. For that purpose, systemic therapies that are selected for you usually begin with drugs that are less toxic while very effective in getting the cancer into control.

There will be certain types of treatments your oncologists will recommend too that are known as **combination therapy**—meaning not just a combination of chemotherapy drugs but a combination of different types of systemic therapies, such as chemotherapy plus a biologic or a biologic plus a PARP inhibitor. Some are pills and others are given intravenously in treating metastatic breast cancer. Sometimes two or more drugs work together to augment each other's actions with few additional side effects. This is especially true of the newer targeted therapies, which oncologists often combine with a traditional chemotherapy drug to enhance their effect.

Combination therapy

Treatment using more than one type of therapy simultaneously.

29. How will the doctor determine if the treatments I am receiving are actually working?

It usually takes two or three cycles of therapy before your oncologist will know if it is working. After two or three cycles, your oncologist will likely repeat your scans to see if your metastases have gotten bigger or smaller. If there are new metastases or the ones that you have now are bigger, your oncologist will likely stop the treatment that you are taking and discuss alternative forms of treatment with you. It does not make any sense to continue with a treatment regimen that is not working. You and your oncologist should be thrilled if the size and number of your metastases are smaller, but you should also be pleased if your cancer is unchanged. Without treatment, metastatic breast cancer progresses, and, after a couple of months, if it is stable, it is probably because the chemotherapy has stopped it from growing. It is quite possible that there will be less cancer the next time your doctor repeats the scans.

"Stable or improved disease" is the definition of success that you and your oncologist should use to assess how well the chemotherapy is working. It sometimes takes a couple of months to see this, and that is why you have to wait before you repeat the scans. However, if it is obvious from your doctor's examination that the cancer is growing at a fast pace, even after one cycle of therapy, there is probably no reason to continue it. You or your oncologist might also stop the therapy if you are having unusually severe side effects.

It is essential that you understand how your oncologist will determine if the therapy is working. You should know when the doctor will make this assessment, and how. It may not always be necessary to do a scan. If, for example, your doctor can feel an enlarged **lymph node** in your neck, she will likely get a scan to see how large it is and if there are other lymph nodes that appear to be containing cancer too. If you have cancer in your liver, your liver function tests may be elevated, and your doctor can follow these to determine if you are responding to treatment. Even in these situations, your oncologist will probably want to repeat scans from time to time, so that she can more fully assess your response to therapy.

In addition to measuring the amount and size of your metastases, your oncologist may also use your symptoms to know whether the therapy is working. If the

"Stable or improved disease" is the definition of success that you and your oncologist should use to assess how well the therapy is working.

Lymph node

Tissue in the lymphatic system that filters lymph fluid and helps the immune system fight disease.

*Your oncolo-
gist will in-
dividualize
your systemic
therapy dose
and schedule
to maximize
the chance that
your cancer
will respond
and minimize
the side effects
that you will
experience.*

therapy makes you feel better, this is usually a sign that it is working. Good clinical signs that the therapy is working include pain that improves with chemotherapy, a poor appetite or weight loss that is now better, or feeling less tired. Some treatments, however, might make you feel worse due to the side effects of the drug(s). Your doctor will determine if you are experiencing side effects from treatment versus progression of the cancer.

In summary, the definition of *working* is when the cancer is not getting any worse. Oncologists generally continue giving therapy as long as it is working or until you have unacceptable side effects. You should expect your doctor to assess these factors every two to three cycles of therapy. Sometimes this assessment is spread out a bit after you have had more therapy.

You should make sure that your doctor has a facility that will meet your needs. It can take anywhere from 1 to 8 hours or more to get your treatment, depending on the type of therapy that you are getting. If your systemic therapy requires IV administration, you will probably get it while seated in a comfortable, reclining-type chair in the chemotherapy infusion center. If you're receiving a different systemic treatment, it still will be given in the same setting as chemotherapy is given. There are beds available in some infusion centers, but you will probably be more comfortable in the specially designed recliners. If there are no TVs at the place where you get your therapy, you may want to bring your own DVD player, laptop, or a book to read. You should dress comfortably, and you may want to bring a snack or light lunch. It may be possible for a family member or friend to keep you company while you get your treatment, but space is usually quite limited and you may want to nap during much of your infusion. Although there is nothing particularly scary about seeing someone receiving therapy, young children are easily bored and should probably stay at home.

30. How is systemic therapy given?

Oncologists give systemic therapy in different ways, depending on the location of your metastases and the drugs that your oncologist gives you. The four most common methods are intravenous, oral, intramuscular, and intrathecal.

The *intravenous* (*IV*) route is the most common way of giving chemotherapy. An oncology nurse inserts a small plastic needle into one of the veins in your lower arm so that the chemotherapy can flow through it. Since a needlestick is required to get into the vein, you may have some minor, temporary discomfort. After that, infusion of the therapy is usually painless. The therapy flows from a plastic bag through the needle and catheter into the bloodstream. Sometimes the oncology nurse uses a syringe to push the chemotherapy through the tubing. Therapy can also be infused into your veins through a **vascular access device (VAD)** also known as an **implantable port**. An implantable port is a hollow disk, about the size of a quarter, that is placed under the skin, usually on the chest wall under the collarbone. To access the device, the nurse inserts a special needle through the skin into the port. If this hurts you, she can apply a numbing cream to the skin before she inserts the needle. A nurse must flush the device once a month to prevent it from clotting. No other care is required between treatments. Since this device is completely under the skin, you can shower and bathe with no worries.

Vascular access device (VAD)

A method of transferring medication directly into a vein or artery.

Implantable port

A disk placed under the skin to allow repeated direct access into a blood vessel.

The *intramuscular* (*IM*) method involves getting an injection directly into the muscle. There is a slight pinch as the nurse places the needle into the muscle of the arm, thigh, or buttocks; however, the procedure lasts only a few seconds. This route is usually not used to give breast cancer chemotherapy, but it is used occasionally to give hormonal therapy.

Intrathecal therapy may be necessary when breast cancer spreads to the nervous system. This usually involves injecting the therapy directly into the spinal fluid after your doctor does a spinal tap.

The *oral* (*PO*) route takes the form of a pill, capsule, or liquid taken by mouth. This is the easiest and most convenient method since it can be done at home. Researchers are working hard to develop new therapies that can be taken by mouth so that you can avoid coming to an infusion center to receive your treatment. Though this is great for giving you more freedom and control over how you spend your time, it requires that you adhere to the treatment regimen as prescribed.

31. What is a systemic therapy cycle?

Oncologists give systemic therapy according to a particular schedule that is based on the type of cancer being treated and the particular drugs being used. Your therapy may be given daily, weekly, every 2 to 3 weeks, or monthly. There are even certain drugs given orally that are given daily for several weeks, then you stop taking it for a specific number of days, and then you resume taking it again. These treatment days are followed by rest days to allow your body time to recover from the effects of the therapy. This schedule of treatment and rest days is called a *cycle*. There usually is no choice on the interval or for how many days of the cycle you will receive the therapy. Your oncologist will decide how many cycles of a given therapy to give you based on how well your cancer responds to treatment and on the side effects that you experience. They may give it for a set number of cycles, but when treating metastatic breast cancer, oncologists usually continue treatment as long as it is working.

You need to be diligent in taking your drugs exactly as prescribed. If it is a somewhat complicated schedule of when you are to take the pills orally, create a written schedule so that you can mark off each time you have taken the medication. Pill boxes designed for taking pills at certain times of the day and on what days can be helpful in keeping you on track. Have a family member help you with this. Your oncologist, nurse practitioner, or nurse navigator may have some helpful tips too. And if you are having side effects, you must report them to your treatment team. Don't delay in doing this. There are likely some things the treatment team can do to help minimize the side effects. Sometimes, however, the dosage of the drug needs to be reduced to see if that helps diminish the side effects. This is okay. Don't assume the drug isn't working if you need to take a lesser dose.

The side effects of therapy depend on the properties of the drug, not on how you take it.

32. How long will I take a particular systemic treatment? Before, when I had an earlier-stage cancer, I took specific drugs for a certain number of cycles or for a specific period of time.

When you were originally diagnosed with an earlier stage breast cancer, the purpose of the systemic treatments you received was to prevent you from getting metastatic disease. You received these treatments as what is called adjuvant therapy. Evidence-based research was used to determine a specific dosage, as well as a specific number of cycles of treatment, that provide the optimal treatment (number of cycles of therapy or a specific length of time) to prevent the cancer from spreading elsewhere in the body. So if a cancer cell had traveled to another organ site like your bones, liver, or lungs, the adjuvant systemic therapy you received was intended to kill any cells that reached these organs. In your case, that didn't work, so now you will be receiving different drugs from those that didn't work before, and you will take them for as long as they are doing their job in keeping the metastatic disease in control. So it is a big change from the purpose of your previous systemic treatment.

33. My doctor just told me that my cancer is in remission. Does that mean that I'm cured? He mentioned a term, NED. What does that mean?

Remission is the word that oncologists use to describe how well the anticancer treatment is working. It is not the same as *cure*. Remissions are *complete* or *partial*. Complete remission means that there is no longer any sign of cancer on your examination, blood work, or scans. This is also known as **NED**, which means there is no evidence of disease on any scans. *Partial remission* means that there is less cancer in your body than there was before treatment but there is still some sign of cancer on your examination, blood work, or scans. Sometimes partial remissions become complete

NED

No evidence of disease on scans.

remissions after you get more treatment. The more cancer the treatment kills, the better, and complete remissions usually last longer than partial remissions. Unfortunately, when it comes to metastatic breast cancer, even complete remissions (NED) are not forever. Though not curable, metastatic breast cancer is usually quite responsive to initial therapy, and there is a good chance that you will enjoy a remission for some time before the cancer grows back.

There are times that you may be doing so well with your scans showing NED that your doctor decides to have you take a drug holiday. This means that you will be off treatment for a period of time, which is always refreshing because your body can kind of reset itself to a more normal state of being. Some patients don't want a drug holiday, fearing that being off treatment for even a short time will trigger the cancer cells to start growing again. This will be something to discuss with your oncologist if a drug holiday is offered.

34. What are my chances of remission, and how long might it last?

That is not an easy question to answer. Some women with metastatic breast cancer live with their disease in remission for years, while others never have a remission and die within months. The likelihood that your cancer will respond to treatment depends on many complex factors. Your overall health and well-being and the amount of metastatic disease are important, but the most important predictor is how well you respond to the first couple of cycles of therapy. Usually, the faster and more complete your initial response, the longer it will last. Every time your breast cancer comes back, the chance of it responding to a new treatment regimen decreases, and the duration of the remission gets a bit shorter. With time, your breast cancer will no longer respond to treatment, and the focus of your care will change to managing the symptoms, often with the help of palliative care or hospice nurses. Although the proper time for this transition is a very personal decision, most oncologists feel that the chances of responding to additional therapy are virtually nonexistent if you have not responded to your last three therapy regimens or if you are spending most of your day in bed or a chair.

The likelihood that your cancer will respond to treatment depends on many complex factors.

Breast cancer that has metastasized to the bone or soft tissues generally grows more slowly, and responds to treatment more completely and longer, than breast cancer that involves the liver, lung, or brain. Breast cancer that recurs after many years generally grows more slowly and responds to treatment better than breast cancer that recurs during, or shortly after, the initial diagnosis and treatment.

35. Since my therapy affects my immune system, is it still okay for me to work while taking it? Are there any precautions I should use in the workplace or in other social settings?

The purpose of any therapy is to allow you to live your life in as normal a manner as possible, for as long as possible. These therapies will certainly affect you, but you should strive to go about your regular business as much as you can. Though these therapies will affect your immune system, this is really only a problem when your white blood cell count is low.

White blood cells (WBC), more specifically, the group of white blood cells called *neutrophils*, fight infection, and, when they are low, you are at increased risk for infection. Your white blood cells drop to their lowest point (**nadir**) in the middle of your cycle of therapy, stay there for a few days, and then gradually increase back to normal. Your greatest risk of infection is, therefore, in the middle of your therapy cycle.

Nadir
The low point of blood counts that occurs as a result of systemic therapy.

It is prudent to minimize your exposure to sources of infections during the entire time that you are on systemic therapy, but this is most important during the nadir period. You do not need to be a hermit during this period, but you should not go out of your way to be around people with colds and fevers. This is easy to do in your own home where you can ask visitors to stay away if they are sick.

This is harder to do at work or in large social settings, especially if you do not want to share your diagnosis with coworkers and friends. You need to be in control of your environment, especially when your WBC count is low. If this is not possible, it is best to avoid these situations all together or, if you must, limit the time of your exposure and wear a mask. It should go without saying that you should not share things like towels or drinking glasses, and always use commonsense hygiene measures like handwashing.

The purpose of any therapy is to allow you to live your life in as normal a manner as possible, for as long as possible.

Actually, most infections that people get during therapy come from the germs that normally inhabit your intestinal tract or skin. Your immune system usually keeps these germs in their own place, but when your WBC count is low, they can sneak through these natural defenses and cause an infection. Over the years, studies have shown that antibiotics, nutritional supplements, or a change in your diet will not prevent this from happening. Fortunately, the majority of patients who get therapy do not get infected, and those who do usually respond to antibiotics quite nicely. However, immediate treatment is critical, and it is very important for you to call your doctor right away if you have a fever or any signs or symptoms of infection—even if these occur at 2 o'clock in the morning!

We do know from a Johns Hopkins employee benefits program called *Managing Cancer at Work*, which is provided to businesses and corporations across the country, that those employees who choose to work while receiving their treatments are happier having made this decision because it provides a means of maintaining a routine, and it diminishes the amount of time they are thinking about their cancer; in addition, their coworkers are likely part of their support team.

Continuing to work is, of course, a personal choice. Some patients need to work for financial reasons or to maintain their health insurance. A nurse navigator and/or social worker can review with you what the human resource policies are that are tied to federal laws that protect your job and you from discrimination and afford you the opportunity to have reasonable accommodations at work. If and when you become sicker and unable to perform your duties, you probably need to consider being at home or working part time. Don't overtax your body when it needs to be working to help keep the cancer in control.

36. My doctor checks my blood count just before I get my next dose of chemotherapy. Why does he also need to check it 1–2 weeks later?

Your blood counts reach their nadir about 1–2 weeks after you get your chemotherapy. After a few days, they start to rise and usually return to normal in time for you to start your next cycle of therapy. Your doctor checks your blood counts on the day that you get therapy (or the day before) so that she will know if it safe for you to start your next cycle of therapy. If your white blood cells or **platelets** are too low, you will probably need to wait until they return to a safe level before you get your next treatment. Your oncologist may also want to know how low your counts get at their nadir. This helps her decide if she needs to modify the dose of your therapy or the interval between your treatments. If your WBC nadir is unusually low, or if you have **neutropenic fever** or infection, your oncologist may decide to give you a cytokine (*Neulasta* or *Neupogen*) the day after your next therapy infusion to try to prevent this from happening again. She also uses these mid-cycle nadir blood counts to advise you on the need for any special precautions or treatments to protect yourself from infection (due to low WBC counts) or bleeding (due to low platelet counts). There are now devices available that give you the freedom of not having to return to the infusion center to get some of these cytokine agents. It self-administers the drug to you using a small device that sticks on your upper arm. One product that does this is called *Neulasta Onpro*.

Platelet

A component of blood that assists in clotting and wound healing.

Neutropenic fever

A fever due to a low white blood cell count, usually caused by a side effect of chemotherapy.

Most infections that people get during therapy come from the germs that normally inhabit your intestinal tract or skin.

37. When I have a problem, should I call my primary care doctor or my oncologist?

That depends on what the problem is. Your cancer or treatment may affect your other medical problems, and it is critical that all of your doctors communicate with each other. For example, the corticosteroids (prednisone or *Decadron*) that oncologists use as therapy premedication, or to help control nausea and vomiting, may make gastric acid problems worse or increase your blood sugar, making your diabetes worse. If you have high blood pressure, your doctor may need to adjust your antihypertensive medicines. Most oncologists prefer that your primary care doctor continue to manage your health issues unrelated to cancer, but since your primary care doctor may not always be aware of some of the problems associated with certain cancers or cancer treatments, it is important that you tell your oncologist about all of your medical problems. For example, the low-grade fever and sore throat that your primary doctor usually tells you to treat with acetaminophen and saltwater gargles may require hospitalization and intravenous antibiotics in the setting of a systemic therapy–induced low WBC count. A good rule of thumb is, when in doubt, call your oncologist's office, and let them decide who should take care of the problem.

38. Is it safe to travel while I am getting my therapy?

Although sticking to the therapy schedule is important, the schedule is not nearly as inflexible as many people think that it is. You will probably be getting systemic therapy for the rest of your life. Since the goal of therapy is to allow you to live your life, it is imperative that you do so, sometimes despite the therapy itself. Holidays, vacations, and family life-cycle events are part of everyone's life. Just because you are getting therapy does not mean that you need to forgo these pleasures. Tell your oncologist when they will occur, and do not be surprised when she accommodates your therapy schedule around those events. Unless it becomes a regular practice, a day here or there or an occasional extra week between cycles will have little impact on how well the therapy works, especially once you have a few treatment cycles under your belt. During your regular cycle of therapy, there are better times to travel than others. The best time to travel is once you are through the nadir period of **cytopenias**, just before you are due to get your next treatment. Also, don't start a new treatment within a few days of traveling or attending an event such as a wedding or graduation because the side effects initially may prevent you from being able to go. Don't allow cancer to have control over you. You need to remain in charge. Document on a calendar when these types of milestone events are scheduled to happen in the coming months, and provide that information to your treatment team. Always make sure that your oncologist knows of your travel plans, and be sure to carry with you a summary of your therapy treatment and latest blood counts. If you do not have access to a doctor through the friends or relatives whom you plan to visit, ask your oncologist to give you the name of a local oncologist in case you run into trouble. Of course, make sure that you take your oncologist's telephone and fax number with you. There may be some countries that your doctor advises you not to visit because of safety concerns. This means they have very limited medical care there or they have a known outbreak of an infectious disease that could seriously harm you. Heed his advice.

Cytopenia

Low cell count (usually in relation to white blood cells).

Since the goal of therapy is to allow you to live your life, it is imperative that you do so, sometimes despite the therapy itself.

PART FIVE

Hormonal Therapy

How does the doctor determine if I should get hormonal therapy and/or CDK4/6 inhibitor therapy instead of chemotherapy?

Are there different types of hormonal therapies? How does my doctor decide which to use?

I am taking hormonal therapy for the treatment of my metastatic breast cancer. Is it true that chemotherapy is better than hormonal therapy because it is given intravenously?

More . . .

39. How does the doctor determine if I should get hormonal therapy and/or CDK4/6 inhibitor therapy instead of chemotherapy?

Hormonal therapy is only an option if your cancer cells have hormone receptors present. When your breast cancer was first biopsied, the pathologists tested your cancer cells to see if estrogen receptors (ER) or progesterone receptors (PR) were present. Unless this test found at least one of these hormone receptors, your cancer will not respond to hormone therapy.

Breast cancers may keep the same hormonal receptor profile forever. However, from time to time, hormone receptor-positive (HR+) cancers become negative. It is unusual for a hormone receptor-negative (HR–) cancer to change to HR+. If your doctor suspects that the hormone receptor status of your cancer may have changed, she may want to biopsy one of the metastatic spots and send it to a laboratory for estrogen and progesterone receptor tests.

If your cancer is not estrogen receptor-positive or progesterone receptor-positive or both, chemotherapy might be used or, depending on your HER2 receptor status (being positive or negative), there may be other therapy options that are specifically designed for type of disease you have. The decision is based on the status of each of the three receptors (ER, PR, and HER2) based on the biopsy done on one of the areas where the cancer has metastasized.

Hormonal therapy is usually the first treatment used in postmenopausal women, unless their tumor is HR–.

Although it may have side effects, those associated with hormonal therapy are usually tolerated much better than the side effects of chemotherapy. Hormone therapy is especially useful in patients whose metastatic disease involves only bone or soft tissue. Though it is also useful in treating metastases to the vital organs (liver, lung, etc.), chemotherapy often works faster in these situations.

40. Are there different types of hormonal therapies? How does my doctor decide which to use?

There are various options your doctor will consider when making decisions about what hormonal therapy to recommend. First and foremost, the cancer cells must be ER+. Then your doctor will consider which type of therapy might work best. There are three general categories of hormonal therapy: Some block ovarian function, others block production of estrogen, and still others block estrogen's effects in the cells.

Blocking Ovarian Function

The ovaries are the main source of estrogen in premenopausal women, so estrogen levels in these women can be reduced by eliminating or suppressing ovarian function, which is called **ovarian ablation**.

Ovarian ablation can be done surgically to remove the ovaries (called **oophorectomy**) or by treatment with radiation. This type of ovarian ablation is usually permanent and may not be the first choice for women who want to have children in the future. However, there

Ovarian ablation

Using surgery or radiation to reduce or eliminate the ovaries' ability to produce estrogen.

Oophorectomy

An operation to remove the ovaries.

are alternatives that are less permanent—drugs called gonadotropin-releasing hormone (GnRH) agonists, also known as luteinizing hormone-releasing hormone (LH-RH) agonists. Some examples of FDA-approved medications for ovarian suppression are goserelin (*Zoladex*) and leuprolide (*Lupron*). Here's how they work: Your ovaries produce estrogen, but the messages that trigger estrogen production are generated in the pituitary gland of the brain in the form of GnRH and LH-RH, so medications that suppress these hormones will also reduce how much estrogen the ovaries produce. It's the equivalent of cutting the power cord or switching off your phone—the messages from the brain telling the ovaries to make estrogen simply won't get through.

Blocking Estrogen Production

Aromatase inhibitor

A drug that suppresses the enzyme aromatase, which the body uses to produce estrogen.

Blocking ovarian function is one way to reduce the amount of estrogen that cancer cells have available. Another way is to use drugs called **aromatase inhibitors**, which block the activity of an enzyme called aromatase that the body uses to produce estrogen in the ovaries and elsewhere. FDA-approved aromatase inhibitors for breast cancer include anastrozole (*Arimidex*) and letrozole (*Femara*), both of which temporarily inactivate aromatase, and exemestane (*Aromasin*), which permanently inactivates aromatase. Aromatase inhibitors are preferred for use in postmenopausal women because in premenopausal women, the ovaries are still actively producing so much aromatase that the drugs cannot keep up—so they're not as effective as we'd want them to be. However, these drugs can be used in premenopausal women if they are combined with a drug that suppresses ovarian function.

Blocking Estrogen's Effects

Reducing the amount of estrogen in the body helps slow or stop tumor growth, but as was mentioned in Question 27, estrogen serves many purposes in maintaining long-term health, particularly with respect to bone strength, so there's a downside to suppressing it. As an alternative, however, pharmaceutical companies have developed several medications that instead interfere with estrogen's ability to attach to estrogen receptors in breast cancer cells, preventing the estrogen from stimulating tumor growth. These medications include the following:

- **Selective estrogen receptor modulators (SERMs)** are drugs that bind to estrogen receptors, preventing estrogen from binding to the tumor cell. One of these, tamoxifen (*Nolvadex*), has been used for more than 30 years to treat HR+ breast cancer. Toremifene (*Fareston*) is another FDA-approved drug in this class. SERMs are different from aromatase inhibitors in that they not only can potentially block estrogen's activity (this is called being an *estrogen antagonist*) in some tissues, but they may also mimic estrogen's effects (which is called being an *estrogen agonist*) in others. For example, tamoxifen blocks the effects of estrogen in breast tissue but acts like estrogen in the uterus and bone.

Selective estrogen receptor modulator (SERM)

A drug that binds to the estrogen receptor. In some tissues (breast), a SERM acts as an estrogen antagonist; in others it acts as an estrogen agonist.

- Other **anti-estrogen drugs**, such as fulvestrant (*Faslodex*), work in a somewhat different way to block estrogen's effects. Like SERMs, fulvestrant binds to the estrogen receptor and functions as an estrogen antagonist. However, unlike SERMs, fulvestrant has no estrogen-agonist effects. It is a pure anti-estrogen. In addition, when fulvestrant binds

Anti-estrogen drug

A drug that suppresses estrogen and damages the estrogen receptor but has no estrogen agonist effects.

to the estrogen receptor, the receptor is damaged and no longer functions, further preventing tumor cells from using estrogen to grow.

Your doctor will determine which of these medications is the best option for you based on the findings of extensive clinical trials that showed which drugs worked best under your specific circumstances, and whether combination with a CDK4/6 inhibitor improves the result.

41. How is hormonal therapy used to treat breast cancer?

There are specific ways that hormonal therapy is used to treat hormone-positive breast cancer:

Adjuvant therapy for early-stage breast cancer: Research has shown that women who receive at least 5 years of adjuvant therapy with tamoxifen after having surgery for early-stage ER+ breast cancer have reduced risks of breast cancer recurrence, including a new breast cancer in the other breast, and reduced risk of death at 15 years.

Tamoxifen is FDA-approved for adjuvant hormone treatment of premenopausal and postmenopausal women (and men) with ER+ early-stage breast cancer, and the aromatase inhibitors anastrozole and letrozole are approved for this use in postmenopausal women. A third aromatase inhibitor, exemestane, is approved for adjuvant treatment of early-stage breast cancer in postmenopausal women who have received tamoxifen previously.

If you were previously treated for breast cancer, you may have received adjuvant hormone therapy to reduce the chance of a breast cancer recurrence. Typically, adjuvant therapy medication is taken every day for 5 years or possibly longer. If you are premenopausal, you may have taken tamoxifen, and if postmenopausal, you may have taken an aromatase inhibitor every day for 5 years, instead of tamoxifen. You may have even received additional treatment with an aromatase inhibitor after 5 years of tamoxifen. It is also possible that you may have switched to an aromatase inhibitor after 2 or 3 years of tamoxifen, for a total of 5 or more years of hormone therapy. Now that you are dealing with metastatic breast cancer, your oncologist will be evaluating what type of hormonal therapy to give you. Part of this will be based on what you have already received and factoring in that it didn't work as intended in keeping metastatic disease at bay.

Several types of hormone therapies are approved to treat metastatic or recurrent HR+ breast cancer. Hormonal therapy is also a treatment option for ER+ breast cancer that has come back in the breast, chest wall, or nearby lymph nodes after treatment (also called a locoregional recurrence).

Two SERMs, tamoxifen and toremifene, are approved to treat metastatic breast cancer. The antiestrogen fulvestrant is approved for postmenopausal women with metastatic ER+ breast cancer that has spread after treatment with other hormonal therapy agents. It may also be used in premenopausal women who have had ovarian ablation.

The aromatase inhibitors anastrozole and letrozole are approved to be given to postmenopausal women as initial therapy for metastatic or locally advanced hormone-sensitive breast cancer. These two drugs, as well as the aromatase inhibitor exemestane, are used to treat postmenopausal women with advanced breast cancer whose disease has worsened after treatment with tamoxifen.

Some women with advanced breast cancer are treated with a combination of hormone therapy and a targeted therapy. For example, the targeted therapy drug lapatinib (*Tykerb*) is approved to be used in combination with letrozole to treat HR+, HER2+ metastatic breast cancer in postmenopausal women for whom hormone therapy is indicated.

Another targeted therapy, palbociclib (*Ibrance*), was granted accelerated approval several years ago for use in combination with letrozole as initial therapy for the treatment of HR+, HER2− metastatic breast cancer in postmenopausal women. Palbociclib inhibits two enzymes called *cyclin-dependent kinases* (CDK4 and CDK6) that appear to promote the growth of HR+ breast cancer cells.

Palbociclib is also approved to be used in combination with fulvestrant for the treatment of women with HR+, HER2− advanced or metastatic breast cancer whose cancer has gotten worse after treatment with another hormone therapy.

Faslodex (fulvestrant) is a type of hormonal therapy medicine used to treat postmenopausal women diagnosed with advanced-stage HR+ breast cancer. Previous research studies had shown that tamoxifen, anastrozole, letrozole, and exemestane worked similarly in slowing or stopping the growth of metastatic breast cancer cells. Research studies have confirmed that administering fulvestrant with a CDK4/6 inhibitor is more effective in slowing or stopping the growth of metastatic breast cancer for ER+, HER2– disease. Premenopausal women with HR+ breast cancers should undergo oophorectomy, either surgically, induced with radiation therapy, or with medicine. Tamoxifen is also an option for premenopausal women whose cancer is HR+ and was not treated with it in the past. If the cancer is in organs other than the bone, the oncologist may decide to be more aggressive with chemotherapy or other treatments to get the cancer to shrink in these organ sites (lung and liver in particular) and then go with more of a maintenance regimen of hormonal therapy.

42. Can other drugs interfere with hormonal therapy?

Certain drugs, including several commonly prescribed antidepressants (those in the category called selective serotonin uptake inhibitors, or SSRIs), inhibit an enzyme called CYP2D6. This enzyme plays a critical role in the use of tamoxifen by the body because it metabolizes, or breaks down, tamoxifen into molecules, or metabolites, that are much more active than tamoxifen itself.

The possibility that SSRIs might, by inhibiting CYP2D6, slow the metabolism of tamoxifen and reduce its effectiveness is a concern given that as many as one-fourth of breast cancer patients experience clinical depression and may be treated with SSRIs. In addition, SSRIs are sometimes used to treat hot flashes caused by hormone therapy.

Many experts suggest that patients who are taking antidepressants along with tamoxifen should discuss treatment options with their doctors. For example, doctors may recommend switching from an SSRI antidepressant such as paroxetine hydrochloride (*Paxil*), which is a potent inhibitor of CYP2D6, to one that is a weaker inhibitor, such as sertraline (*Zoloft*), or that has no inhibitory activity, such as venlafaxine (*Effexor*) or citalopram (*Celexa*). Or they may suggest that their postmenopausal patients take an aromatase inhibitor instead of tamoxifen.

Other medications that inhibit CYP2D6 include the following:

- Quinidine, which is used to treat abnormal heart rhythms
- Diphenhydramine, which is an antihistamine
- Cimetidine, which is used to reduce stomach acid

People who are prescribed tamoxifen should discuss the use of all other medications with their doctors.

If your cancer has recurred while you were taking adjuvant hormonal therapy, your doctor may prefer to switch to a different hormonal therapy, and it may be combined for CDK4/6 inhibitor therapy if the metastatic breast cancer is HER2–. This initial treatment for your metastatic breast cancer, known as first-line therapy, is a common treatment, particularly if your cancer is limited to the bone. Another option may be to switch to a different type of hormonal therapy than you were using when the cancer was discovered as having spread.

Chrissie's comments:

It frustrates me that I'm only receiving hormonal therapy right now for the treatment of my recently discovered metastatic disease. I want it cut out, killed with chemo, and zapped away with radiation. That makes sense to me. The doctors say that less aggressive treatment may get it into control—that is the mission now. I still think that the mission is to be cured. I need to start thinking of this disease as a chronic disease, and that is hard to do.

43. I am taking hormonal therapy for the treatment of my metastatic breast cancer. Is it true that chemotherapy is better than hormonal therapy because it is given intravenously?

No. Many cancer patients make the mistake of thinking that medicine given in the veins is more powerful than medicine given by mouth. This is not true. Hormonal therapy can actually be more effective than intravenous chemotherapy in a woman whose tumor expresses hormone (estrogen or progesterone) receptors, especially when her metastatic disease is confined to the bones or soft tissue.

While hormonal therapy is usually given by mouth or IM injection, some medicines are not absorbed into the bloodstream through the gastrointestinal tract, so doctors have to administer it directly into the bloodstream through a vein. It does not really matter how the anti-cancer medicine gets into your body, as long as it does.

Another common misconception about cancer therapy is to assume that the severity of its side effects is directly related to its anti-tumor strength. Just because a treatment is toxic does not mean that it is effective, and

Different types of hormonal therapies are used to treat cancer in post-menopausal women from those used in pre-menopausal women.

the lack of toxicity does not correlate with inactivity. Unfortunately, many cancer treatments are associated with debilitating side effects, but their anticancer effect relates to how the cancer cells respond to the drug, not how it affects your normal cells.

Many cancer patients make the mistake of thinking that medicine given in the veins is more powerful than medicine given by mouth.

44. I have osteoporosis. Is it safe to take an aromatase inhibitor?

Although aromatase inhibitors (anastrozole, letrozole, and exemestane) are usually the hormonal treatments of choice in postmenopausal women with metastatic breast cancer, they may cause problems for women with osteoporosis, such as worsening bone loss and increased fracture risk. In contrast, fulvestrant is the first type of endocrine treatment that works as an *estrogen receptor downregulator*. This means that it binds to the estrogen receptor site in competition with estrogen in the body. Once it binds to the site, it can cause the receptor to break down, thereby preventing the normal cellular response to estrogen. It has no agonist effects, however, which means that it is bone friendly—a side effect for other hormonal therapy drugs that are part of the aromatase inhibitor drug group. Yet, having osteoporosis does not mean that a woman cannot use an aromatase inhibitor. Rather, these women do need to have their osteoporosis managed aggressively and followed closely.

Osteopenia

A condition of less bone density or bone mass than would be normally expected if you compare a woman to a woman or a population of women her age. It is the bone loss that, if it continues, can lead to osteoporosis.

All women should have a bone density study (DEXA scan) before starting an aromatase inhibitor. If you are not already doing so, you should take appropriate calcium citrate and vitamin D3 supplements. If you have been taking these supplements regularly, and your bone density scan shows significant **osteopenia** or osteoporosis, you should start taking oral bisphosphonates, such

74

as alendronate sodium (*Fosamax*), risedronate sodium (*Actonel*), or ibandronate sodium (*Boniva*). If you have osteopenia but have not been taking calcium citrate and vitamin D3, it is reasonable to try these supplements first. By following your bone density on repeated DEXA scans, your doctor can see if these oral therapies are working. Most insurance companies will pay for only one DEXA scan a year; this is usually adequate in this situation.

If these measures do not work, intravenous bisphosphonates, such as zoledronic acid (*Zometa* or *Reclast*) given two to three times per year, may allow you to remain on an aromatase inhibitor. On the other hand, if you have no major risk factors like blood clots, you and your doctor may want to consider switching to tamoxifen. It is still an excellent drug for breast cancer, and it has less risk of aggravating your osteoporosis. If you are prone to falling or have already had a broken bone due to osteoporosis, you should probably simply avoid the aromatase inhibitors altogether.

PART SIX

HER2–Positive Biologic Targeted Therapy

What does "HER2" actually mean? Does having it mean my cancer is genetic and might be passed down to my kids?

How does the pathologist determine if my cancer cells are HER2–positive or HER2–negative?

What is biologic targeted therapy, and how does it work?

More . . .

45. What is HER2–positive breast cancer, and how do I know if I have it?

Each normal breast cell contains the *HER2* gene, which helps normal cells grow (more about this in Question 46). This gene, also called *HER2/neu* or *cERB-b2*, is found in the DNA of a breast cell. This gene contains the information for making the HER2 protein receptor on the cell's surface. In normal cells, the HER2 protein receptor helps send growth signals from outside the cell to the inside of the cell. These signals tell the cell to grow and divide.

Some breast cancer cells have an abnormally high number of *HER2* genes per cell. When this happens, too much HER2 protein appears on the surface of these cancer cells ("overexpression"). Thus, HER2+ cancers are those that overexpress the HER2 protein receptor. This overexpression of the HER2 protein causes cancer cells to grow and divide more quickly.

Approximately 25% of breast cancer patients have HER2+ tumors. It is very important for you and your doctor to know if your breast cancer is one of these. If it is, your treatment program will most likely contain a monoclonal antibody that blocks the effects of the growth factor receptor protein HER2 (see Question 49).

46. What does "HER2" actually mean? Does having it mean my cancer is genetic and might be passed down to my kids?

HER2 actually stands for "human epidermal growth receptor 2"—but knowing that doesn't really tell you what the *HER2* gene does. The *HER2* gene is a normal gene that everyone has in healthy breast cells. Its job is to direct the production of special proteins that are called HER2 receptors. Each healthy breast cell contains two copies of the *HER2* gene, and as mentioned in Question 45, the function of the *HER2* gene is to help control how cells grow, divide, and repair themselves.

In normal cells, the HER2 protein combines with other proteins to transmit growth signals from outside the cell to the center of the cell. If the growth signal is strong, the cell gets the message to subdivide and create new cells. But now and then, DNA reproduces itself incorrectly, and if a cell has too many copies of the *HER2* gene because of this kind of mistake, it can result in too much of the HER2 protein being produced. In cancer cells with too much *HER2*, a growth signal is continuously being sent from the HER2 protein, resulting in cells subdividing more rapidly than they should. This may result in the normal breast cell turning into a cancer cell—so in that sense, HER2+ cancer is genetic, in that it's caused by a **mutation**, or mistake in DNA.

However, the *HER2* gene, also known as an oncogene, is totally different from the *BRCA1* and *BRCA2* breast cancer gene mutations that are associated with genetic reasons why someone developed breast cancer. *BRCA1* and *BRCA2* gene mutations can be (and are) passed from one generation to another, but the defective DNA containing extra *HER2* genes generally isn't. And the *HER2* genes themselves aren't defective or misbehaving. They behave as intended—there are just too many of them. So think of *BRCA1* and *BRCA2* gene mutations as being associated with hereditary breast cancer. HER2 is a prognostic feature of a breast cancer cell and is not something passed along

Mutation

A change or error in a gene. Specific mutations have been linked with breast cancer.

genetically within a family. So you may have HER2– breast cancer and your mother had HER2+ breast cancer. You both may carry the *BRCA1* gene mutation.

47. How does the pathologist determine if my cancer cells are HER2–positive or HER2–negative?

Immunohisto-chemistry (IHC)

The most commonly used test to see if a tumor has too much of the HER2 receptor protein on the surface of the cancer cells. The IHC test gives a score of 0 to 3+ that indicates the amount of HER2 receptor protein. It also measures the presence of hormone receptors on the breast cancer cell and determines if a tumor is hormone receptor-positive or -negative.

Fluorescence in situ hybridization (FISH)

This is a lab test that measures the amount of a certain gene in cells. It can be used to see if an invasive cancer has too many *HER2* genes. A cancer with too many of these genes is called HER2 +.

Tests performed by the pathologist on the invasive cancer cells help determine whether the *HER2* gene in those cells is normal or abnormal. This testing is known as an oncogene measurement. If the HER2 test is "positive" (sometimes recorded on the pathology report as being "+++" or "3 plus"), then it means that the cancer cells have too much HER2 receptor protein on the surface of the cell or there are extra copies of the *HER2* gene that can stimulate the cells to create too many abnormal cells. This can lead to the production of more breast cancer cells, as well as determining how aggressive those cancer cells are.

The pathologist has two approved methods for testing the HER2 receptors: **immunohistochemistry** or IHC (known as the DAKO HerceptTest) and **fluorescence in situ hybridization** or FISH (Vysis PathVision). IHC measures the HER2 receptors on the surface of the tumor cells obtained from a biopsy. If the number is higher than normal, the tumor is said to be overproducing the HER2 protein. The results of this test are reported as 0, 1+, 2+, or 3+. If the result is 3+, then the breast cancer is considered HER2+. If the result is a score of 2+, it is considered borderline, and the tumor cells should be retested by the FISH method. A finding of 1+ or 0 means the tumor is HER2– and would not be expected to respond to HER2 targeted therapy.

The FISH test detects the presence of too many copies of the gene. This means that the cancer cells have the capacity to make too much of the HER2 receptor protein, making the cancer cells in some cases less likely to respond to certain types of treatments.

It is understandable that it is confusing, given that a test showing positive numbers does not necessarily mean that the final prognostic value is positive—and may actually be negative.

48. How is HER2 different from other prognostic factors?

Prior to understanding the actual biology of HER2+ disease, treatments had been limited to cutting it out (surgery), burning it (radiation), and the use of chemicals (chemo and hormonal therapies). It took a long time to solve the mystery behind this type of breast cancer biology, but the research into the *HER2* oncogene and its receptor finally resulted in the development of ways to treat the disease in a targeted manner based on its biology.

A great deal of research over the past 25 years has been focused on the presence of HER2 receptors and how they help to predict how well a patient is going to do if her HER2 test is positive versus negative. As a result of this research, it has been proven that a HER2+ cancer may mean that the breast cancer is a bit more mischievous than those that are HER2–. A HER2+ cancer grows more rapidly and has a higher incidence or recurrence in the future. Initially, these research findings were frightening to patients whose breast cancer was HER2+. That has changed as a result of this research, however, because new drug therapies have been created specifically for patients whose breast cancers are HER2+, like yours. It also opened the doors and paved the way for the development of treatments designed to biologically alter the cells as a way of treating the disease for early-stage breast cancer and control the disease for stage IV breast cancer, which you now have.

In many cases, for women with HER2+ breast cancers, biologic targeted therapy likely was recommended as part of your adjuvant therapy when you were diagnosed with an earlier stage of breast cancer in the past. Being able to alter the behavior of cells is key to the future of increasing longevity, reducing mortality, and making treatment in the long run easier to accomplish for women diagnosed with HER2+ metastatic disease today as well as potentially other stages in the future.

49. What is biologic targeted therapy, and how does it work?

In recent years, scientists have made great strides in understanding the complicated biological pathways that cause cancer to develop, grow, and spread. They use these drugs because they block specific **biological pathways**—which is basically shorthand for the complex interactions among hormones and proteins within a cell that cause changes in the cell and in tissues—and proteins involved in the growth and spread of cancer.

Biological pathway

The complex interactions among hormones and proteins within a cell that cause changes in the cell's behavior.

Drugs that target the hormone receptors (ER and PR, as discussed in Part 5) found on many breast cancer cells are among the oldest forms of breast cancer treatment.

Drugs like tamoxifen and fulvestrant block the estrogen receptor so that the cancer cells cannot get enough fuel and the cancer cells die. Other anti-estrogens, like the aromatase inhibitor anastrozole, decrease the amount of estrogen in postmenopausal women by blocking the aromatase enzyme needed to make estrogen. But these drugs work differently from the biologic targeted therapies because the targeted therapies are "smart drugs" that focus on molecular and cellular changes that are specific to cancer. Hormonal therapies can't discriminate between receptors on a tumor and receptors in normal breast tissue or even normal tissue outside the breast; for this reason, targeted cancer therapies may be less harmful to normal cells and more effective than traditional hormonal therapies or chemotherapy.

Drugs that target the hormone receptors (ER and PR) found on many breast cancer cells are among the oldest forms of breast cancer treatment.

Many of the biologic targeted therapy drugs block specific enzymes or growth factor receptors (GFRs) found on many cancer cells. Biologic targeted therapy really works in three different ways: it may block tumor cell growth; it may target the cell for destruction by the immune system itself; or it may work with chemotherapy to destroy the HER2+ breast cancer cells. This is truly your body's immune system being given the ammunition it needs to fight your cancer by destroying it as well as preventing it from continuing to thrive. The targeted therapies used to treat metastatic breast cancer include trastuzumab (*Herceptin*), lapatinib (*Tykerb*), neratinib (*Nerlynx*), and olaparib (*Lynparza*).

Monoclonal Antibodies

Trastuzumab (*Herceptin*) is a type of targeted therapy called a **monoclonal antibody** that was the very first drug developed specifically for HER2+ breast cancer. It works by taking advantage of the body's basic mechanism for dealing with harmful intruders. In response

Monoclonal antibody
A medication that targets antigens in specific cell types or tissues.

83

Antigen

A foreign substance that may be a threat to the body—for example, chemicals, virus particles, bacterial toxins, or cancer.

Antibody

A special protein produced by your immune system to help protect the body from disease.

to foreign substances called **antigens** that may be a threat to the body—for example, chemicals, virus particles, bacterial toxins, or cancer—the immune system produces a type of protein called an **antibody**. Each type of antibody is unique and defends the body against one specific type of antigen. Because an antibody binds only to a specific antigen, it can act as a homing device to a tumor cell. The term *monoclonal* means it is derived from one specific type of cell—in this instance, a breast cell. Monoclonal antibodies may be able to kill tumor cells themselves, or they may be linked with tumor-killing substances in a "piggyback" system that allows treatment substances, such as drugs or radioactive materials, to be delivered directly to the tumor. Because the HER2 protein transmits growth signals to breast cancer cells, trastuzumab is an active drug in the 25% of breast cancer patients who have too much HER2 (see Questions 45–47). In metastatic breast cancer, trastuzumab can be given as a single agent, but it is usually used initially with traditional chemotherapy drugs like paclitaxel.

Kinase Inhibitors

If you were initially diagnosed with HER2+ breast cancer at an earlier stage of breast cancer, you likely received trastuzumab as part of your prior adjuvant therapy. You might also have received the drug neratinib (*Nerlynx*), which would have been given to you after you completed a year of taking trastuzumab. Neratinib has been used in the adjuvant setting to prevent metastatic disease from occurring in HER2+ patients who were considered at high risk for developing metastatic disease, and it is also approved for treating metastatic disease after it occurs. Your doctor may be discussing neratinib with you now, as a new option for managing HER2+ metastatic breast cancer.

From a technical perspective, neratinib is known in the biological world as a *kinase inhibitor*, which requires a bit of explanation. Human cells have many different enzymes called kinases that help control important functions, such as cell signaling, metabolism, division, and survival. Certain kinases are more active in some types of cancer cells, and blocking them may help keep the cancer cells from growing. Kinase inhibitors may also block the growth of new blood vessels that tumors need to grow; like any other tissue, cancer needs a good blood supply to survive.

Immune Checkpoint Inhibitors

An important part of the immune system is its ability to distinguish between normal cells in the body and those it sees as "foreign." This lets the immune system attack the foreign cells while leaving the normal cells alone. To do this, it uses "checkpoints"—molecules on certain immune cells that need to be activated (or inactivated) to start an immune response. Cancer cells sometimes find ways to use these checkpoints to avoid being attacked by the immune system. But new drugs that target these checkpoints hold a lot of promise as cancer treatments. These will be discussed further in Question 54.

Other Adjunct Targeted Therapies

It is exciting to see more drug options becoming available for patients with HER2+ metastatic disease.

Lapatinib (*Tykerb*), for instance, is a small molecule that inhibits HER2 proteins. Because it has a different mechanism of action than trastuzumab, lapatinib is useful in patients with HER2+ breast cancer whose breast cancer has progressed following treatment with standard chemotherapy agents such as doxorubicin (*Adriamycin*) or epirubicin (*Ellence*), targeted therapy agents such as neratinib, taxane agents such as nab-paclitaxel (*Abraxane*) or docetaxel (*Taxotere*), and trastuzumab. Unlike trastuzumab, lapatinib is an oral drug. It is usually given in combination with capecitabine (*Xeloda*), another standard chemotherapy drug.

More recently, a class of drugs called PARP inhibitors has been developed. These drugs will be discussed in greater detail in Questions 50–53 where we look at HER2– cancers, but they can also be used in HER2+ cancers. One such drug, olaparib (*Lynparza*), is approved for patients who have already received trastuzumab as part of their adjuvant therapy to reduce the risk of distant recurrence.

50. I have HER2–negative metastatic breast cancer. Does that mean I have only toxic chemotherapy or possibly hormonal therapy to help me?

In the past, the answer would have been "yes," but today, as a result of laboratory research and clinical trials, there are now more options for women who have HER2– metastatic disease. The drugs we mentioned in the preceding question, the PARP inhibitors olaparib (*Lynparza*) and talazoparib (*Talzenna*) have been approved to treat advanced-stage HER2– breast cancer in people with a *BRCA1* or *BRCA2* gene mutation.

PARP stands for poly (ADP-ribose) polymerase, which is an enzyme that fixes DNA damage in both healthy and cancerous cells. Research has shown that medicines that interfere or inhibit the PARP enzyme make it harder for cancer cells with a *BRCA1* or *BRCA2* mutation to fix DNA damage. This means a PARP inhibitor makes some cancer cells less likely to survive the DNA damage done by conventional treatments, like chemotherapy drugs.

51. How long can I stay on a PARP inhibitor?

Just as in the case for other treatments that you will be receiving, your oncologist will do blood tests and scans to determine how effectively these treatments are working for you. As long as they are helping you and you are tolerating side effects well, then you will continue on this therapy until it isn't working for you as it once did.

It is important to offer this therapy to patients likely to benefit from it. Someone originally diagnosed with hormone receptor-positive breast cancer should have been either prescribed some form of hormonal therapy or else determined not to be a candidate for it for other medical reasons before they can be considered for this type of treatment. PARP inhibitors are given to patients who have previously been treated with chemotherapy. This form of treatment is a pill taken by mouth and has been deemed the first nonchemotherapy for treating patients who are HER2– and carry a breast cancer gene mutation.

52. How will I know if I carry one of the BRCA gene mutations? Is genetic testing part of my routine blood work?

Genetic testing is definitely not part of the routine blood work that you currently are having done. This test looks at your genes to determine if a cancer-related mutation is present. From the perspective of standard of care, all patients with stage IV breast cancer are to be genetically tested due to the availability of PARP inhibitors to provide an additional way to get and keep the cancer under control. Such a test involves testing either your blood or your saliva. The test is sent away to a laboratory that is designed for genetic testing. It usually takes about 2 weeks for the results to come back.

Ideally, you would meet with a genetics counselor or other genetics expert to receive education and counseling about what the test results may mean and what the likelihood is that you carry such a gene mutation. Your family history is very important here, so take the time to talk to family members and inquire who in your ancestry has had some form of cancer and specifically what kind it was, back three generations. This may not be as easy as it sounds; years ago, people didn't talk about cancer and definitely not about breast cancer. They may have said something like, "Grandma had a 'female problem' that made her very weak, and she died from it." Well, that doesn't tell you much—you need specifics!

Pay close attention to the mention of breast, ovarian, pancreatic, or prostate cancer under the age of 60, as well as melanoma. These types of cancers are linked together on *BRCA1* and *BRCA2* gene mutations. *BRCA1* is linked to ovarian and breast cancers, and *BRCA2* has been connected to breast, ovarian, and pancreatic cancer, melanoma, and prostate cancer occurring at a relatively young age. These two mutations are the most common, but there are also other gene mutations associated with breast cancer that the genetics expert will review with you and for which you'll be tested.

Counseling is important because genetics testing has other ramifications. The genetics counselor or expert will create your family **pedigree**—a family tree that includes information on which family members have had what types of cancers. From this, along with some additional information about your own breast cancer, he or she will be able to interpret whether it is likely you have a gene mutation. The obvious hope is that knowing that you have a gene mutation will provide you with additional treatment options. However, a positive result also would mean that your biological siblings and offspring may carry the same gene mutation that increases their risk of the specific types of cancers referenced above. The likelihood is pretty significant, as 50% of siblings and 50% of offspring would carry the same gene mutation you have.

Pedigree

A family tree that documents different kinds of cancers occurring within your family, usually three generations back.

An individual must be of legal age to be tested, which could prevent underage children or siblings from finding out if they have the mutated gene. Discovering who is positive and who is negative can stir up sibling rivalry, guilt, or resentment. Parents also can experience feelings of guilt when it is determined who among them carried this gene mutation, since no one wants to hand down a cancer-causing gene to his or her child. So there are a lot of repercussions arising from this test.

53. If I carry a gene mutation, should my whole family be tested?

The idea of testing everyone in your family once you've had a positive result is actually a bit of a slippery slope. Family members would benefit from meeting with the genetics counselor, at least among those who are of legal age. They need to each decide personally if they want to be tested. Not everyone does. Some people prefer not to know; others want to know everything and do everything to reduce their risk of getting one of these types of cancers. For example, if you had a sister who also carried the same gene mutation, she may choose to have her ovaries and fallopian tubes taken out along with doing bilateral mastectomy with reconstruction. But a sister who hasn't finished birthing her family may choose to wait to take action until some time in the future. Men get tested too because, although their risk of getting breast cancer is low (6% for those who carry a gene mutation), they need to be mindful of the other cancers, too, that aren't manageable preventively. Being part of a high-risk genetics program can help with closer monitoring.

54. What exactly is immunotherapy, and might I be a candidate to receive it at some point too?

Immunotherapy medicines work by helping your immune system work harder or smarter to attack cancer cells. The immunotherapy medicine atezolizumab (*Tecentriq*) is an immune checkpoint inhibitor, which means it targets a specific protein that helps cancer cells hide from the immune system—in this case, the protein PD-L1. PD-L1 is a protein extending from the cancer cell surface that allows some cells to escape an attack by the immune system. PD-L1 interacts with a protein called PD-1 on important immune system cells called T cells. This coupling—known as an **immune checkpoint**—instructs the T cell to leave the tumor cell alone. Checkpoint inhibitor drugs prevent the PD-1/PD-L1 meeting from taking place. Without

Immune checkpoint

A connection between the PD-1 protein on T cells and PD-L1 protein on cancer cells that causes the immune system to ignore the cancerous cell rather than kill it.

receiving the "stop" signal from the PD-L1 protein, the T cells can go ahead an attack the tumor cells.

A PD-L1 test, which involves sending a piece of tumor tissue to a lab for analysis, helps doctors determine whether a patient is likely to benefit from immune checkpoint inhibitors like atezolizumab. By inhibiting PD-L1, atezolizumab essentially allows immune system cells to "see" the cancer cells and kill them. Atezolizumab is used in combination with the chemotherapy medicine nab-paclitaxel (*Abraxane*) as the first treatment for locally advanced or metastatic triple-negative, **PD-L1–positive breast cancer** that can't be removed surgically.

PD-L1–positive breast cancer

Breast cancer that contains the PD-L1 protein, which prevents immune cells from killing the cancer.

PART SEVEN

Side Effects of Metastatic Breast Cancer and Its Treatment

What kinds of side effects might I expect to experience as a result of getting treatment for my metastatic breast cancer?

My chemotherapy and hormonal therapy have caused me to develop symptoms of menopause. How can I manage these symptoms and feel more like myself again?

I am feeling more joint pain and backaches that make it difficult to walk around. What can I do to manage my pain?

More . . .

55. What kinds of side effects might I expect to experience as a result of getting treatment for my metastatic breast cancer?

There are various side effects that a patient may experience while receiving treatment for metastatic disease, as well as symptoms of progression of disease, that warrant discussion with your doctor. Some are easily controlled, and some may be more difficult. No two patients are alike, so if you knew someone with metastatic disease in the past, don't assume that your situation will mirror theirs.

In the questions that follow, I explain some of the more common side effects. You should discuss these with your oncology team so you know what to expect in relation to the status of your metastatic disease and the treatment recommendations they are making on your behalf.

These questions are not intended to alarm you but to provide you with a comprehensive list of possible issues that may need to be addressed while you are undergoing treatment. There is also a section called Breast Cancer Drug Therapy Information toward the end of this book that provides you with more details about potential side effects associated with each drug. Remember that just because a drug may have a side effect listed, it doesn't mean you will definitely experience it. But if you do, speak up, so interventions can be taken to diminish it or even totally obliterate it.

Marissa's comments:

The side effects from chemo and hormonal therapy were really getting to me. My most miserable problem was night sweats that prevented me from sleeping well. I found that installing a ceiling fan above my bed and keeping it on low all night really helped. Wearing short-sleeve and sleeveless cotton nightgowns instead of pajamas that were long sleeved with long pants has been a godsend too. I even found a thing called a "chillow pillow" online that keeps my head feeling cool all night. This makes dealing with these symptoms from treatment a lot more tolerable and doable long term now.

Jill's comments:

I attended a support group provided by the hospital where I'm receiving my treatments. It is for breast cancer survivors, but most of the women who were attending were diagnosed early and were completing treatment or had finished treatment long ago. They were fussing and moaning about their hair growing back slowly or having hot flashes still. This group was not for me, and I told the social worker who was the facilitator so. I finally found a group that was specifically for women with metastatic breast cancer. We are all in the same situation—some with disease that is very advanced and others with disease that is more stable, but the bottom line is we share the same worries, fears, and hopes. I can relate to these women.

56. Why do I feel so tired most of the time? Is there anything I can do to get my energy back?

Feeling exhausted or extremely tired is probably the most common side effect patients report. This can happen as a side effect of chemotherapy and/or radiation therapy. Approximately 70% of patients with advanced cancers report this as a frustrating chronic symptom.

If there are specific problems you are experiencing that are related to fatigue, such as difficulty sleeping, make your doctor aware so that he might prescribe something for you to help. Ask about how to better manage your pain, if that is a contributing factor. Also ask about coping with your emotional distress, which can increase fatigue. Fatigue can also be triggered by anemia, so it's important that you mention it to your doctor so he or she can rule out this possibility (see Question 62 for more on anemia).

Conserving your energy is important so you have what you need to spend time doing things that are important to you. Make a list of the activities and chores you are trying to accomplish, and see about recruiting family and friends to assist you. You may also notice that your energy is better during certain times of the day. The Oncology Nursing Society has a website that provides some specific recommendations related to managing this treatment side effect. Take a look at www.cancersymptoms.org/symptoms/fatigue/. Also visit the National Comprehensive Cancer Network's website for more information at www.nccn.org.

57. I've heard that some drugs can damage the heart. Is this true?

There are several drugs that can produce a side effect of heart problems: Doxorubicin (*Adriamycin*), which is a chemotherapy agent, trastuzumab (*Herceptin*), and biologic targeted agents in the CDK4/6 inhibitor family can cause heart problems too. Even long after you have finished trastuzumab, for example, you can develop heart problems related to the drug's cardiotoxicity.

Your doctor will use a **MUGA scan** or an **echocardiogram** to help determine if it is safe to give these medications. The MUGA or echocardiogram may be repeated every few months to reevaluate the heart's functioning and ensure that all is well and that it is safe to continue with your treatment. Congestive heart failure, a weakness of the heart muscle, can occur but is not common. These risks are greater when trastuzumab or doxorubicin are given together. Some women are given trastuzumab alone with a very low risk to their heart. If you experience shortness of breath or chest pain, you need to report it to your oncologist right away so a determination can be made whether it is caused by a drug you are receiving or if it is related to your cancer, which may cause breathlessness due to a buildup of fluid in the lung area (**pleural effusion**; see Question 63) or pain if the cancer is pressing on a nerve (see Question 61). Tests can be done to determine the underlying cause, and from there, your doctor can go ahead and treat the reason these symptoms are happening.

MUGA scan

A special heart X-ray that determines the strength of the heart.

Echocardiogram

A special test using ultrasound that determines the strength of the heart.

Pleural effusion

Excess fluid that accumulates in the pleural cavity, the fluid-filled space that surrounds the lungs. This excess fluid can impair breathing by limiting the expansion of the lungs.

58. My chemotherapy and hormonal therapy have caused me to develop symptoms of menopause. How can I manage these symptoms and feel more like myself again?

Approximately 40% of women dealing with breast cancer develop menopausal symptoms from breast cancer treatments. This can be an issue particularly for women who are premenopausal and are undergoing chemotherapy and/or hormonal therapy for control of their disease. These symptoms are thought to be caused by a decline in estrogen and other hormones and can include hot flashes, night sweats, vaginal dryness, pain during intercourse, difficulty with bladder control, insomnia, and depression. Some patients use **complementary therapies** such as vitamins, soy products, or black cohosh to try to reduce symptoms. Currently, there are no studies to give us definitive answers about the use of these supplements. It is worth talking to your doctor about his thoughts if you wish to consider taking any.

Some patients find that taking a medication like venlafaxine (*Effexor*) can be helpful in reducing hot flashes. Wearing cotton clothing in layers that can be peeled off as needed also can be a useful measure on your part. There are various vaginal lubricants that can be used for vaginal dryness and pain during intercourse. These include Replens, Astroglide, or K-Y Jelly. Avoid using petroleum-based products (petroleum jelly), as they can increase risk of vaginal infections. Avoid spicy foods, smoking, alcohol, caffeine, hot showers, and hot weather, all of which can trigger hot flashes.

59. I'm taking so many different medications now that my stomach is always upset. What can I do to feel better and be able to eat and enjoy food again?

Nausea and vomiting are relatively common side effects associated with chemotherapy drugs. With the development of anti-nausea medicines (called **antiemetics**), the incidence of nausea and vomiting has reduced considerably. When beginning new medications, such as hormonal therapy, these side effects may be problematic for

Complementary therapy

An intervention used in conjunction with standard therapies.

Antiemetic

A drug used to stop or prevent nausea or vomiting.

a while. Pain medications have a reputation for contributing to nausea, too. Severe nausea that interferes with your ability to eat or retain foods can cause dehydration. Changes in what you eat and drink may be useful in managing nausea and vomiting.

Some specific suggestions include:

- Eat a light meal before each chemotherapy treatment.
- Have small amounts of food and liquids at a time.
- Have bland foods and liquids.
- Eat dry crackers when feeling nauseated.
- Limit the amount of liquids you take with your meals.
- Maintain adequate liquids in between meals; drink mostly clear liquids, such as water, apple juice, herbal tea, or bouillon.
- Eat cool foods or foods at room temperature.
- Avoid foods with strong odors.
- Avoid high fat, greasy, and fried foods.
- Avoid spicy foods, alcohol, and caffeine.
- Suck on peppermint candies to help reduce or prevent nausea.
- Rub peppermint-flavored lip balm above your lips and below your nose so that you are smelling mint, which may reduce nausea.

If these strategies aren't helping, ask your oncologist for a prescription for an antiemetic, and ask if you can take it in a preventive manner to prevent, reduce, and control nausea. These medicines include such drugs as ondansetron (*Zofran*), granisetron (*Kytril*), and prochlorperazine (*Compazine*). When loss of appetite is severe,

Peripheral neuropathy

Numbness and pain of the hands and feet, which can be caused by infection, very strong drugs (such as chemotherapy), or disease.

sometimes an appetite-stimulant drug called megestrol (*Megace*) is prescribed.

60. My feet and hands have gotten tingly. What is this, and how can I make it go away?

Neurological problems, such as **peripheral neuropathy**, are possible side effects of some chemotherapy drugs. Peripheral neuropathy is damage to peripheral nerves—that is, the nerves in your hands and feet. There are three types of peripheral nerves: sensory, motor, and autonomic. Sensory nerves allow us to feel temperature, pain, vibration, and touch. Motor nerves are responsible for voluntary movement and allow us to walk and open doors, for example. Autonomic nerves control involuntary or automatic functions such as breathing, digestion of food, and bowel and bladder activities. When there is damage to the peripheral nerves, the symptoms depend on the types of peripheral nerves affected. Though chemotherapy drugs can affect any of the peripheral nerves, the most common ones affected are the sensory nerves, causing numbness and tingling in the hands and feet. In patients who already have peripheral neuropathy from other causes—for example, diabetes—chemotherapy can sometimes make it worse.

Symptoms of peripheral neuropathy include:

- Numbness and tingling, which may feel like pins and needles in your hands and/or feet
- Burning pain in your hands and feet
- Difficulty writing or buttoning a shirt
- Difficulty holding a cup or glass
- Constipation

- Decreased sensation of hot or cold
- Muscle weakness
- Decreased hearing or ringing in the ears (known as tinnitus)

If you develop any of these symptoms, it's important to tell your doctor right away. Describe the symptoms you are experiencing. If you already have any of these symptoms before starting chemotherapy, tell your doctor. Your doctor may decide to prescribe medication for you to reduce these symptoms. The medicines most commonly used are drugs that are given to neurology patients for treatment of seizures and depression. Some examples are gabapentin (*Neurontin*), carbamazepine (*Tegretol*), and amitriptyline (*Elavil*). Additional measures you should consider taking at home include paying close attention when you walk and avoid having scatter rugs in your house. Keep your home well lit so you can see where you are walking. If you are still driving a car, be sure you can feel the foot pedals. If temperatures are hard to decipher, then ask for help in checking the temperature of the bathwater as well as any hot beverages you are drinking. Take extra precautions to guard against frostbite in the winter. Some patients have had effective relief by seeing a cancer rehabilitation therapist, so inquire about that option too.

61. I am feeling more joint pain and backaches that make it difficult to walk around. What can I do to manage my pain?

For some patients, pain may be the most difficult symptom to cope with and overcome. Metastatic breast cancer that has spread to the bones, for example, can cause bone pain that is very uncomfortable (see Question 70). It can reach a point of making it difficult to walk around and function well because the pain is so intense. A primary goal for you and your doctor is to prevent pain from being debilitating if it happens. Your doctor will prescribe pain medications for you.

Sometimes it takes several different types of medications to get pain under control. This is usually more of an issue for patients toward the end of life. If you're taking narcotics for pain management, avoid driving, as your alertness may be impaired, and you may be more prone to accidents. Some pain medications can cause constipation, so talk with your doctor about taking stool softeners to prevent bowel problems.

The goal is for pain to be manageable and not so uncomfortable that your quality of life is negatively affected. Tell your doctor if the pain medications are no longer working as well as they did when first prescribed. Adjusting medications is a continuous and expected process.

62. What is anemia, and how is it treated?

Red blood cell (RBC)

A type of cell in the blood with the primary function of carrying oxygen to tissues.

Hemoglobin

The part of the red blood cell that carries the oxygen.

By definition, anemia is an abnormally low level of **red blood cells (RBCs)**. These cells contain **hemoglobin**, which provides oxygen to all parts of the body. If RBC levels are low, parts of the body may not be receiving all the oxygen they need to work and function well. In general, people with anemia commonly report feeling tired. The fatigue that is associated with anemia can seriously affect quality of life for some patients and make it difficult for patients to cope at times.

Anemia is a common problem for many dealing with cancer. It is especially an issue for those undergoing chemotherapy. Medications such as epoetin (*Procrit, Epogen*) or darbepoetin (*Aranesp*) may be recommended to stimulate your bone marrow to make more red blood cells, raising your blood cell count and increasing your energy level. Such a medication is given by injection under the skin using a very small, thin needle. The doses vary and it is common to be given one of these medications for this side effect once a week. You might be advised to also take an oral iron supplement while getting these injections.

The fatigue that is associated with anemia can seriously affect quality of life for some patients and make it difficult for them to cope at times.

63. My metastatic breast cancer spread to my lungs, and I've noticed it is getting harder to breathe. Why might this be?

Fluid around the lungs, or pleural effusion, is a condition that presents commonly as shortness of breath, dry cough, a feeling of heaviness in the chest, inability to exercise, and a feeling of being unable to take a deep breath. This is due to extra fluid building up around the pleural spaces of the lungs. A malignant pleural effusion is caused by cancer cells that grow into the **pleural cavity**. Many patients with metastatic breast cancer develop this problem.

Pleural cavity

A space between the outside of the lungs and the inside wall of the chest.

The diagnosis of pleural effusion is made by physical examination and chest X-ray. Treatment is based on the amount of fluid in your chest and if you have any symptoms. If the fluid collection is considered to be large and you have noticeable symptoms, the doctor may decide to insert a needle through the ribs into the pleural space and remove the fluid. Sometimes this is done with the

Thoracentesis

The removal of fluid from the pleural cavity through a hollow needle inserted between the ribs.

Pleurodesis

A procedure that gets rid of the open space between the lung and the chest cavity.

help and guidance of ultrasound. This procedure is called a **thoracentesis**. It can be done on an outpatient basis.

Sometimes the fluid comes back, and you will need to have it drained again. If this happens frequently, your doctor may suggest a procedure called **pleurodesis**. This is done to stop fluid from building up in this space. When cancer cells are growing in this space, they make fluid that can collect and cause difficulty breathing. During this surgery, a chemical is placed in the space. Your body's reaction to the chemical causes the lining around the lung to stick to the inside lining of the chest wall.

Sitting up and using pillows for support can sometimes make breathing easier. Reclining chairs may be more helpful for sleeping than trying to lie flat in bed. Supplemental oxygen may be given as well to help with breathing. If oxygen is given at home, great care must be taken. The use of matches, cigarettes, or candles is not allowed in the room where the oxygen is in use or being stored, because pure oxygen is highly flammable. Oxygen containers should be kept far away from gas or electrical heating elements, too. The respiratory therapist or company that provides the oxygen will review other safety measures with you and your family or caregivers.

64. I have been prescribed Lynparza for my metastatic breast cancer, and I was told that I need to avoid drinking fruit juices, which I love. Why is this a requirement of taking this medicine?

There are specific types of juices that you need to discontinue taking because they affect how your body processes the medication. Grapefruit, grapefruit juice, Seville oranges, and Seville orange juice may increase the level of Lynparza in your blood. So, to ensure that you're getting the dosage that is prescribed, avoid these fruits and juices during treatment. Grape juice is fine, however.

65. What can I do to manage hair loss?

The technical term for hair loss is **alopecia**. The hair on your head falls out, and if hair on other parts of your body (such as eyelashes or eyebrows) grows rapidly, it may fall out too. Alopecia is a relatively common side effect of several chemotherapy agents used to treat and manage breast cancer. You may have already experienced this when you had your initial breast cancer treatment. For women needing radiation to their brain, hair loss can happen again and may occur in a few areas or all over, depending on how the radiation was given.

Alopecia
Hair loss.

Hair loss has become a signal that the person is a cancer patient. It can be psychologically and physically difficult to cope with hair loss since it is associated with our self-image, womanliness, health status, and other personal issues related to how we feel about our hair.

Getting a wig in advance of hair loss can be helpful so that your hairstyle, texture, and color can be matched well for you. Some insurance companies cover the expense of a wig. Check your policy and see if your insurance company covers "skull prosthesis for side effects of cancer treatment." Costs that are not covered are tax deductible. There are programs like "Look Good, Feel Good" that most cancer centers offer to their patients. This is a special program available free of charge to show you how to wear turbans, scarves, and makeup to reduce the obvious appearance of hair loss. Ask your

Alopecia is a relatively common side effect of several chemotherapy agents used to treat and manage breast cancer.

doctor or nurse when the facility where you are getting your treatment is offering this program.

Some women actually choose to make a statement and not cover their head at all. It is a personal choice. However, during cold months of the year, you really need to have a head covering that will keep you warm because people lose 80% of their body heat from the top of their head. You should also be careful to avoid sunburn.

66. My doctor mentioned that he would check my calcium levels periodically. What is this for?

Hypercalcemia

Accelerated loss of calcium in bones, leading to elevated levels of the mineral in the bloodstream with symptoms such as nausea and confusion.

Hypercalcemia is an unusually high level of calcium in the blood. There are situations in which it can be life threatening, and it is usually associated with a problem with metabolism caused by the cancer. It occurs in 10 to 20% of people with cancer. Symptoms that would trigger your doctor to check your blood level for this side effect include loss of appetite, nausea, weakness, frequent urination, excessive thirst, feeling confused and unable to concentrate, abdominal pain, or constipation. If the calcium level is very high, it can trigger irregular heartbeat, kidney stones, and loss of consciousness and coma. Intravenous bisphosphonates (zoledronic acid or pamidronate) medications help control this side effect (see Question 71).

67. It seems harder to fight off colds and flu viruses than it did before. How come?

When harmful bacteria, viruses, or fungi enter the body and the body is not able to fight back to destroy these cells on its own using the immune system, an infection develops. Breast cancer patients are at higher risk of developing an infection because the cancer present in their bodies, along with the treatments being given, can weaken their immune systems. Spiking a high fever; chills; sweating; sore throat; mouth sores; pain or burning during urination; diarrhea; shortness of breath; a productive cough; or swelling, redness, or pain around an incision or wound are all symptoms that an infection may be present. To help reduce risk of infection, stay away from young children who may be carriers of flu viruses, colds, and other respiratory illnesses. Though they can look relatively healthy, young children may be harboring germs. This doesn't mean you have to abandon seeing your children or grandchildren, though. It does mean evaluating how the child is feeling and being vigilant for any symptoms, such as a runny nose, fever, or cough, that would signal to you that this isn't a good day to have the child sitting on your lap. Family members who live with you or you see frequently should get flu vaccinations to help reduce the risk of unknowingly bringing viruses your way.

At the first sign you may be getting an infection (fever, cold, etc.), notify your doctor so he can prescribe something for you.

68. My dentures aren't fitting right and have caused ulcers on my gums. What caused this?

This is known as **mucositis**, or mouth sores. It is an inflammation of the inside of the mouth and throat and can result in painful ulcers. Medications like steroids may increase the risk of developing an infection

Breast cancer patients are at higher risk of developing an infection because the cancer present in their bodies, along with the treatments being given, can weaken their immune systems.

Mucositis

A condition in which the lining of the digestive tract, from the mouth to the anus (mucosa) becomes swollen, red, and sore. For example, sores in the mouth can be a side effect of chemotherapy.

in your mouth. Keep your mouth clean and moist to prevent infection. Brush your teeth with a soft-bristled toothbrush after each meal, and rinse regularly. Avoid commercial mouthwashes that contain alcohol because they can irritate the mouth. If you wear dentures that do not fit properly, you will be more likely to get sores in your mouth from rubbing and irritation. This can be a particular problem if you have experienced or are experiencing weight loss, because your gums may shrink, changing the fit of your dentures. See your dentist for an evaluation. If you have dental needs that have not been taken care of prior to starting chemotherapy, ask your oncologist and dentist to talk on the phone and discuss what strategy to use to reduce risk of infection and mouth sores while receiving your treatments.

69. I am about to start treatment with Nerlynx and read that diarrhea is a common side effect. I want to remain as active as possible. How can I manage to do this?

Any time a new drug therapy is started, it is important to sit down with your oncologist, nurse practitioner, and/or nurse navigator and get well educated on the side effects to be aware of, as well as when they might occur. It is usually best to plan not to travel, even the short distance to the grocery store, when first beginning a new treatment regimen like this. Make sure your treatment team knows what your normal bowel habits are, especially if you usually go several times a day. Medications for getting diarrhea under control can be prescribed so you have something to take if diarrhea begins to get out of control. By being home in your own environment (and your own private bathroom), you can take the time for your body to get adjusted to this new treatment. Don't get discouraged or frustrated early on if you have frequent trips to the bathroom. Your treatment team will give you specific instructions about what point to take the prescribed anti-diarrheal medication as well as when to call them urgently if needed. By lightening your schedule so that your body can adjust to this new treatment regimen, it allows you to cope better with the early-onset side effects rather than trying to find a clean restroom out in public somewhere.

70. How will my doctor control my bone pain?

Bone metastases are the most common cause of pain in patients with metastatic breast cancer. Not everyone with cancer in the bones has pain. Radiation therapy is particularly effective in treating bone pain. You may not experience its full effect until a few weeks after the last treatment, so be patient. In the meantime, you should not hesitate to take the pain medicine (**analgesics**) that your doctor prescribes. If you need narcotic medications to control your pain, your doctor may also want you to take a **nonsteroidal anti-inflammatory drug (NSAID)** to make it work better.

Analgesic
A drug that reduces pain.

Nonsteroidal anti-inflammatory drug (NSAID)
A class of pain medication, often sold over the counter, that includes ibuprofen and similar common painkillers.

Of course, the best way to ultimately control and prevent bone pain is for your cancer to go into remission from systemic therapy. Since radiation can make the side effects of chemotherapy worse (especially bone marrow suppression, mucositis, and diarrhea), your oncologist often holds off giving you chemotherapy during the radiation treatments. Your doctor may also recommend radiation therapy to prevent you from breaking a bone,

Nerve block

An anesthetic injection that stops nerve impulses for pain relief.

Vertebroplasty

A procedure to relieve pain from fractures or compression of the vertebrae, in which a special cement is injected into the fractured bone.

even if the cancer in your bones is not causing pain. Intravenous bisphosphonates, such as pamidronate (*Aredia*) or zoledronic acid (*Zometa* or *Reclast*), also help control bone pain and speed bone healing. Be sure to request a referral to a palliative care specialist whose sole focus is on pain management and symptom control. They often can come up with additional therapies that work effectively but aren't therapies your medical oncologist may be familiar with, such as **nerve blocks** or **vertebroplasty**.

71. Is it true that the bisphosphonates that I take for my bones will damage my jaw?

Osteonecrosis

An abnormal die-off of previously healthy bone cells, often in the jaw.

Osteonecrosis of the jaw is a painful disorder caused by loss of blood to the bone tissue and eventual collapse of the jawbone. Recent reports have linked it to the use of intravenous bisphosphonates, but it appears to occur in very few breast cancer patients who are given intravenous bisphosphonates for their bone metastases. The risk is increased in patients who have received prolonged doses of intravenous bisphosphonates, especially in conjunction with chemotherapy and corticosteroids. Additional risk factors include a history of jaw trauma, dental surgery, periodontal (gum) disease, or dental infections. For that reason, doctors recommend that you have a good dental exam with preventive dentistry intervention before you start intravenous bisphosphonate therapy. You should also try to avoid dental procedures during your treatment.

Most oncologists feel that the benefits of intravenous bisphosphonate treatments far outweigh the minimal risk of jaw osteonecrosis. Though it does not affect overall survival, intravenous bisphosphonate infusions significantly decrease skeletal events (fractures, pain) in breast cancer patients who have bone metastases. Either pamidronate (*Aredia*) or zoledronic acid (*Zometa*) is effective, but zoledronic acid is probably slightly better. In addition, it can be infused over 15 minutes and is, therefore, more convenient to get than pamidronate, which has to be given over 2 to 3 hours. Both drugs are given in the outpatient setting every 3 to 5 weeks.

Your doctor may want you to take calcium citrate and vitamin D3 while you are getting these treatments. She will also measure your blood calcium, phosphorus, and magnesium levels at periodic intervals to make sure that they are normal. The bisphosphonates can adversely affect your kidneys, especially zoledronic acid, and your doctor will need to monitor your kidney function with blood tests. Both zoledronic acid and pamidronate are also used to lower the amount of calcium in patients with too much calcium in the blood (hypercalcemia) caused by metastatic breast cancer (see Question 66).

It is smart to get your routine dental prevention and screening exams before and during the time you are taking these medications. If any major dental work needs to be done, get it done before you start this therapy. Also, make your oncologist aware if you have dental implants.

72. How will my doctor treat the swelling and pain that I have in my abdomen?

If your cancer spreads to the lining of your abdomen (peritoneum) you may develop ascites. Just like a child's

Ascites

A buildup of fluid in the abdominal cavity.

bruised knee weeps fluid, tumors irritate the peritoneum and cause it to weep. The fluid that collects in the abdominal cavity is called **ascites**. It may cause swelling, pressure, and pain. The best way to control ascites is with systemic anticancer therapy, but your doctor may also use diuretics (water pills) and pain pills. Occasionally, your doctor may put a needle into your abdomen (paracentesis) to remove some fluid, but this is only a temporary solution since the fluid usually comes back within days to weeks.

73. My partner and I have enjoyed an active sex life. Since my treatments have gotten more intense, this has been more difficult. What can we do to be able to still be sexually intimate? We both miss it.

The percentage of women dealing with metastatic breast cancer who are experiencing problems continuing sexual activity isn't clearly known. Even for the general population of women not dealing with anything as serious as metastatic breast cancer, 43% have reported problems with sexual activity. Some patients find it very difficult to comfortably discuss this issue with their doctor, though it may be very important to their quality of life. Side effects from treatment may result in decreased libido because of hair loss, weight gain, fatigue, or other symptoms, and you simply don't feel well enough to try or confident enough with your self-esteem to engage in sexual activity.

Physical intimacy is one aspect of a loving relationship. It gives us personal pleasure and creates a feeling of closeness to our partner. Sexual intercourse is just one way of being physically intimate. Cuddling, hugging, touching, rubbing, and holding hands are all pleasurable ways of showing one another affection. Talk with your partner about your concerns and feelings. This will help both of you to know how to help each other. Experiment with different positions. You may find one to be more comfortable than another when having sex. Vaginal lubricants can help with vaginal dryness (see Question 58). Some women who have not had success with vaginal lubricants have tried egg whites for lubrication. Be sure to wash thoroughly after intercourse, but do not use douche solutions. If lack of energy impairs sexual activity, plan ahead for intimacy by identifying when you are feeling higher levels of energy during certain times of the day or week. Vaginal discharge, burning, or itching may be signs of a vaginal infection. See your gynecologist if you develop these symptoms so they can be properly treated.

Sexual intercourse is just one way of being physically intimate. Cuddling, hugging, touching, rubbing, and holding hands are all pleasurable ways of showing one another affection.

74. I am so worried about pain. What can be done to avoid it?

When patients are asked the question, "What are you most worried about?", they express a fear of being in pain with no way to get it into control and effectively managed almost 99% of the time. This is why palliative care is important. The priority and sole purpose of palliative care is symptom management.

Palliative care specialists are different from oncologists. They spent time in medical school getting extra training so that you won't be in pain and can continue to experience some joys in your life right up until the end of life. Unfortunately, medical oncologists primarily use opioids for pain control and don't get the palliative care team involved, as they should. Palliative care specialists will try to alleviate the cause of the pain rather than just buffering it with narcotics. Be sure to request a consultation with a palliative care specialist before pain or any of the other side effects discussed in this section begin. This individual, who also is a medical oncologist by training, can learn about you as a person and start the dialogue with you about what your concerns are, and what is important to you and will ask other questions such as

- How much do you know about your cancer?
- How much do you want to know about your cancer?
- What are you hoping for?
- What are you most worried about?
- Tell me three things that bring you joy (or brought you joy before you became sicker)

The palliative care specialists will create a plan to restore or preserve your quality of life. They are amazing. It must be a priority for you to have a consultation with such a professional and remain in touch regularly throughout your journey. They are most involved during the latter half of your journey but can be instrumental early on as well.

Keep in mind, too, not everyone with metastatic breast cancer has pain. However, if you do have pain, rest assured that your doctor will do whatever is needed to control it. You will want to remain as active as possible, however, so drugs that cause you to sleep around the clock are likely not what you will want.

The cancer itself does not cause pain. People with metastatic disease experience pain if the tumor presses on surrounding organs or nerves. One of the major goals of systemic treatment is to control pain, but it may take a couple of months for it to be effective. While you are waiting for this, you will need specific anti-pain treatment. Sometimes the treatment does not kill enough cancer cells to make the pain go away completely, and you will have to continue to take pain medication.

Doctors use medicines and radiation therapy to control pain. The medicines are usually given by mouth, but they are sometimes administered in the veins or by placing medicated patches on the skin. Nerve blocks are often useful in controlling pain that is in a localized area. Relaxation techniques, massage, and acupuncture also have roles in managing some types of cancer pain.

But rely the most on your palliative care doctor. Remember, he is your quality-of-life coach throughout your journey.

PART EIGHT

Clinical Trials

What is a clinical trial? Am I still a candidate to participate in one if I have metastatic breast cancer?

What questions should I ask the doctor about a specific clinical trial she has recommended for me?

How do I find out about clinical trials that might be appropriate for me to consider?

More . . .

75. What is a clinical trial? Am I still a candidate to participate in one if I have metastatic breast cancer?

There are many different kinds of clinical trials. They range from studies focusing on ways to prevent, detect, diagnose, treat, and control breast cancer to studies that address quality-of-life issues.

Most clinical trials are carried out in phases. Specific details about the different phases are found in Question 76, but basically, each phase is designed to learn different information and build on the information discovered previously.

As far as being a candidate is concerned, the short answer is yes—metastatic breast cancer patients may be eligible for Phase I, Phase II, or Phase III studies. The criteria for whether a study will accept a particular patient depends on her stage of disease (some studies are specifically looking at stage IV breast cancer, which is what your metastatic breast cancer is called; others look at various stages including, or excepting, stage IV), what therapies she has already had, and whether specific therapies are planned for her treatment (such as surgery). Patients are closely monitored at specific intervals while participating in studies.

Jessica's comments:

Participating in a clinical trial was important for me because I realize that by doing so, not only am I potentially benefiting myself but also may be helping to establish the new treatment options for women who come after me.

76. What are the various study phases of clinical trials?

Phase I studies are used to find how much of a new drug can be given safely. In such studies, only a small number of patients are asked to participate. When other treatments are no longer working to control your metastatic breast cancer, you may become a candidate to participate in such a trial. The option is offered to patients whose cancer cannot be helped by other known treatment modalities. Some patients have received benefits from participation, but most have experienced no benefits in fighting their cancer. Those who participate in phase I studies are paving the way for the next generation, which is important. Once the optimum dose is chosen, the drug is studied for its ability to shrink tumors in phase II trials.

Phase II studies are designed to find out if the treatment actually kills cancer cells in patients. A slightly larger group is selected for this trial, usually between 20 and 50 patients. Patients whose breast cancer has no longer responded to other known treatments may be offered the chance to participate in this type of trial. Tumor shrinkage is measured, and patients are closely observed to measure the effects the treatment is having on their disease. Some patients may benefit from participation in phase II studies and others may not.

Phase III studies usually compare standard treatments already in use with treatments that appeared to be effective in phase II trials. This phase requires large numbers of patients to participate, usually thousands. Patients are normally **randomized** for the treatment regimen they

There are many different kinds of clinical trials. They range from studies focusing on ways to prevent, detect, diagnose, treat, and control breast cancer to studies that address quality-of-life issues.

Randomized

Describes the process in a clinical trial in which animal or human subjects are assigned by chance to separate groups that allow for comparison of different treatments.

will be receiving. These studies are seeking the benefits of longer survival, better quality of life, fewer side effects, and fewer cases of cancer recurrence.

Supportive care studies are tailored to improve ways of managing side effects caused by treatment. They also include some quality-of-life studies as well.

You may be a candidate for clinical trials in any of these categories, so ask your doctor about clinical trials and see what studies you may qualify to participate in. Over time, you may actually participate in several.

You may derive substantial benefit from participating in clinical trials. Every successful cancer treatment being used today started as a clinical trial. The patients who participated in these studies were the first to benefit. Hopefully, you will be in the next group of patients to benefit from clinical trials that are presented to you for consideration.

77. What questions should I ask the doctor about a specific clinical trial she has recommended for me?

Ask your doctor the following questions:

- What is the purpose of the study?
- How many people will be included in the study?
- What kinds of tests and treatments take place during the study?
- How are treatments given, and what side effects might I expect?

- What are the risks and benefits of each protocol?
- What are the alternatives to the study?
- How long will the study last?
- What type of long-term follow-up care is provided for those who participate?
- Will I incur any costs? Will my insurance company pay for part of this?
- When will the results be known?
- How will you determine if this study is specifically benefiting me, if that is the goal?
- If I'm not alive to hear the final results of the study, how can my family learn about the results of the study if they are interested?

This last question is a tough one to ask, because obviously the hope is that the drugs they are using will enable you to live in harmony with your breast cancer and survive a long time.

There are some studies that are intended for participation after the patient has passed away. An example of such a study is the "Rapid Autopsy Program." It may be hard to imagine having such a clinical trial discussed with you, but it was a very significant study that provided answers as to how breast cancer spreads from the breast to other organs and how it goes about sometimes changing its prognostic factors, such as changing from being hormone receptor-positive to hormone receptor-negative or HER2+ to HER2−. Women who participated in this trial agreed to have tissue harvested upon their death from the organs to which the cancer was known to have migrated, as well as having other organs removed that were thought to be cancer free.

This enabled researchers to study the tissue and learn the process whereby breast cancer travels and changes its features, becoming somewhat of a chameleon. This study resulted in enough new information to allow researchers to develop better treatments for women with metastatic disease. My institution, Johns Hopkins, had 21 women with stage IV breast cancer who agreed to participate; from them, we learned that approximately 22% of the time, one of the prognostic factors of the metastatic lesions did in fact change from what it had been originally in the breast tumor itself. The ultimate goal of the research is to be able to prevent the breast cancer from being able to ever leave the breast in the first place. If this can one day be achieved, then virtually no one would develop metastatic breast cancer and, in turn, no one would die of it. This part of the research effort is still ongoing; such a trial obviously doesn't benefit the patient herself, but it can make a huge difference for the next generation of women who come after her.

Each woman who gallantly participated in this study did so as part of her own personal legacy. I felt humbled as I met with each patient to discuss the study, bringing with me the pathologist who would be doing the autopsy (tissue harvest) procedure. The pathologist spent about an hour with each patient, in my presence, to hear her life story and to also answer any questions she had about the procedure itself. Normally, patients very rarely meet the pathologist who reviews their case. Pathologists prefer staying behind the scenes. But this study brought two people together for a common goal. It is but one example of a clinical trial, but it's probably the most profound clinical trial I have ever known or been a part of.

78. How do I find out about clinical trials that might be appropriate for me to consider?

You can get information from your doctor, but you can also do some homework yourself. Visit the following websites for more information:

National Comprehensive Cancer Network (NCCN) at *www.nccn.org*. You can also use this website to find a cancer center in your geographic region. Contact the center to see if there are any available clinical trials for individuals with metastatic breast cancer. Some trials may be specific for women with stable disease, and others may be for patients who have disease progression.

National Cancer Institute at *www.cancer.gov /clinicaltrials/* or call 800-4-CANCER.

National Institutes of Health at *www.clinicaltrials .gov*. Select "focused search" button and type in "metastatic breast cancer."

Coalition of National Cancer Cooperative Groups at *www.cancertrialshelp.org* or call 877-520-4457.

Centerwatch also provides a list of clinical trials at *www.centerwatch.com*.

Consider also asking the cancer center where you are getting your treatment or getting a second opinion if they have a clinical trials nurse whose job is to match new patients, as well as those coming for a second opinion, with appropriate trials for which they may be a candidate.

The ultimate goal is to be able to prevent the breast cancer from being able to ever leave the breast in the first place.

PART NINE

Complementary and Alternative Medicine

What are complementary and alternative treatments?

I want to try some complementary therapies while receiving my current and future systematic treatments. How do I go about deciding which therapies to try?

Where can I get credible, up-to-date information about research studies that have been done on complementary and alternative medicine?

More . . .

79. What are complementary and alternative treatments?

Complementary and alternative medicine (CAM) is also sometimes referred to as integrative medicine and covers a wide variety of approaches and techniques with the goal of improving health and treating disease. These treatments are not recognized as standard of care or part of conventional treatment by the traditional medical community. When such treatments and methods are used with conventional treatment they are usually referred to as complementary; when used instead of traditional treatment, they are considered to be alternative.

80. I've heard that some alternative medicine treatments may actually cure cancer. Is this true?

There are lots of websites that claim something works. They may be reporting anecdotal evidence or findings from poorly constructed studies conducted by a company to support its product, rather than credible studies that are evidence-based and conducted in the rigid manner in which clinical trials are required to be carried out. These claims sound wonderful and even imply that the product is a "cure for breast cancer," when there may be nothing that scientifically supports those claims. Be cautious of advertisements that, for a fee, claim that the company will mail you the "cure" for your cancer. If what they were selling really was a cure, then an NCI-designated cancer center would be investigating it or offering it—and they'd be the ones telling you about it.

That said, there are some alternative therapies that *might* offer benefits to cancer patients—not in curing cancer, but in helping relieve symptoms. More and more scientifically based research is being done now, and some therapies have been proven to be beneficial for cancer patients. The U.S. government founded the National Center for Complementary and Alternative Medicine (NCCAM) as part of the National Institutes of Health with the intended goal of providing information about what is safe and effective regarding these types of therapies.

It can be difficult, sometimes, to conduct evidence-based medicine clinical trials on these methods of treatment because there may not be clear-cut measurements that can tell us how effective they are in an isolated manner. For example, someone may be doing some form of complementary medicine while also getting a standard treatment. How do you determine which did what? Ask your doctors for their input regarding information you have read about or heard so you can weed out accurate information from claims that may not be correct.

There are some types of therapies that would interfere with the treatments your doctor has given you. For example, certain vitamins in high doses may impair the effect of some chemotherapy drugs. There are other types of therapies that your doctor may encourage you to do, such as **acupuncture**, exercise, or yoga. There are evidence-based research studies supporting these three types of complementary therapies that have demonstrated their benefit to breast cancer patients. Reducing the side effect of nausea, increasing a patient's energy level, and reducing emotional stress have been proven to be clinical outcomes from these types of therapies.

Acupuncture

The technique of inserting thin needles into the skin at specific points. This technique is a form of ancient Chinese medicine and can help control pain and other symptoms for some individuals. It is a form of complementary therapy.

Ask your doctors for their input regarding information you have read about or heard so you can weed out accurate information from claims that may not be correct.

81. What are examples of some complementary and alternative treatments that I might hear about or want to learn more about?

Complementary and alternative medicines may be categorized in many different ways. The NCCAM divides these therapies and treatments into five categories:

1. **Alternative medical systems of theory and practice**. Some of these are traditional healing practices used by various Native American tribes or other cultures. Acupuncture originated as a part of traditional Chinese medicine. Other examples of alternative medical systems are homeopathic and naturopathic medicine.

2. **Mind–body interventions**. These are techniques that aim at helping the mind to enhance various body functions and reduce symptoms. Examples include relaxation, **meditation**, guided imagery, hypnosis, prayer, and support groups.

3. **Biological-based therapies.** These include dietary (for example, a macrobiotic diet), herbal (for example, saw palmetto), biological (for example, shark cartilage), and orthomolecular (for example, vitamins) treatments.

4. **Manipulative and body-based methods**. These are techniques that involve manipulation or movement of the body, such as those used by chiropractors and massage therapists.

5. **Energy therapies.** These are techniques that manipulate energy fields within or outside of the body, such as therapeutic touch, Reiki, or magnets.

The use of complementary and alternative therapies is rapidly increasing. This is partly due to our increasing

Meditation

A mental technique that clears the mind and relaxes the body through concentration.

desire to help ourselves and utilize more natural methods of treating and preventing disease. There is valuable, science-based information about some forms of CAM that confirm some are useful. It is also felt that an increased use of complementary and alternative therapies is a sign that may represent the personal feelings of desperation that many people feel when dealing with metastatic disease. It means we are perhaps willing to try anything and everything that we feel may help us.

It's important to remember that complementary and alternative therapies (specifically supplements or herbals) are not regulated in the same manner that medications and medical devices are. Some pills you see that claim to do certain things may not do anything or potentially may even be harmful to you. For example, some herbal supplements have been found to contain ingredients not listed on the label—including some that are "spiked" with conventional medications as a way of supporting their claims of efficacy! While the companies that do this clearly are not ethical, it can be hard to distinguish the good from the bad. An ethical company will voluntarily comply with the FDA's current good manufacturing practices and will include a label stating that they are "CGMP certified." This tells you that what they say is in the product is actually what's *in* the product.

82. I want to try some complementary therapies while receiving my current and future systemic treatments. How do I go about deciding which therapies to try?

Discuss your thoughts on this with your doctor and inform him that you want to try some complementary therapies. Many, like yoga and prayer, can be done and are safe to use with standard treatments. If you have read about a particular therapy that interests you, bring that information with you to your doctor for his review so that he understands your interest and what you are hoping to accomplish by engaging in this therapy. Therapies that may raise questions about safety and benefit are biological treatments, in particular. Keep in mind that even herbs and vitamins may do you harm in some cases. Because it is available over the counter and may be something you have been taking for years, doesn't mean it is safe to do now. For example, certain vitamins taken in pill form, like vitamin C, can cause certain types of chemotherapy drugs to not work—like the problematic fruit juices described in Question 64, they can change the way a medication is metabolized by your body. This is why it's important to tell your doctor or nurse *everything* you're taking, even multivitamins and herbal teas. So be sure to discuss with your doctor what you were taking before you were diagnosed and what you want to continue taking or consider taking going forward. Concealing from your doctor what you have chosen to do can be a mistake and cause you harm rather than do you good.

83. My disease is progressing and I'm running out of options for treatment. Can I embark on alternative medicine and do it on my own?

It is a patient's right to be able to do whichever treatments she desires, whether her oncologist agrees with her or not. There are some patients who take the alternative medicine road right from the start and refuse any form of standard traditional treatment for their metastatic breast cancer. Although things may seem fine initially, eventually the disease begins to pick up more speed in spreading to other organ sites within the body, and the clinical outcome in these situations isn't good. It is much harder to get control of breast cancer if it involves multiple organ sites and is growing fast.

There may be a point, after traditional treatment has been exhausted and control of the disease is no longer possible, when patients will embark on other routes of treatment on their own. Your doctor should understand this, but he or she will also want you to have realistic expectations. The chance of its helping is small, and the objective is for it not to hinder you in living your life as best you can. The power of the mind should never be underestimated. If we believe we are benefiting from something, then we may be getting a real result. It will be relieving for everyone when more scientifically based research is completed and published to better guide us as to what is wise to do and what may not be in the future.

It is a patient's right to be able to do whichever treatments she desires, whether her oncologist agrees with her or not.

Your doctor and the rest of the treatment team will want to help and support you throughout your journey, including as you transition into deciding to discontinue treatment or add a selection of treatments you want to try on your own. As the cancer advances, oncologists are usually more willing to discuss alternative therapies too. This isn't necessarily because they think the treatments will work but because they know that it is important to you to leave no stone unturned.

It usually is not wise to leave the country for some treatment that you have heard about elsewhere. Your health status usually cannot endure it, it may be incredibly expensive, and it will likely not provide you with what you are hoping for. If and when there are scientifically proven treatments developed elsewhere that become standard of care everywhere, then it will be part of care provided to you here. Even if you hear or read online that such research has been done elsewhere, if it wasn't published in a peer-reviewed medical journal, then it wasn't really evidence-based research. It can be tough to hear, when you become enthused that there is a cure somewhere that you just have to fly around the world to get, that this option likely is not going to benefit you.

There are also scammers out there looking to prey on individuals like you. There is no regulation of what is placed on the internet, so anyone can make up anything and publish it online, or for that matter even write a book about it. That's very unfair to patients like you. So be leery of such claims. If it sounds too good to be true, it usually is.

84. Where can I get credible up-to-date information about research studies that have been done on complementary and alternative medicine?

It is important to have the latest information because this is an ever-changing area of study. The following websites provide good, reliable information:

Cancer Information Services of the National Cancer Institute at *www.cancer.gov/cancerinfo/treatment/cam.*

National Center for Complementary and Alternative Medicine of the National Institutes of Health at *www.nccam.nih.gov/health.*

Memorial Sloane–Kettering Cancer Center at *www.mskcc.org/aboutherbs.*

M. D. Anderson Cancer Center at *www .mdanderson.org/topics/complementary.*

American Academy of Medical Acupuncture at *www.medicalacupuncture.org* or 323-937-5514.

The following sources provide information specifically on dietary supplements, including vitamins, minerals, and botanicals:

Office of Dietary Supplements of the National Institutes of Health at *www.dietary-supplements .info.nih.gov.*

Center for Food Safety and Applied Nutrition of the U.S. Food and Drug Administration (FDA) at *www.cfsan.fda.gov.*

American Botanical Council at *www.herbalgram.org.*

The **National Library of Medicine** at *www.nih .gov/nccam/camonpubmed.html* offers scientific bibliographic citations related to particular therapies.

85. How do I decide if I should or shouldn't use one of the complementary or alternative therapies my family and friends are recommending?

First, do your homework and learn more about the therapy before jumping in and trying it, particularly if it involves taking a product of some type. Some specific questions to think about are:

- Do the promises sound too good to be true? Is here conflicting information about how beneficial this therapy is and its actual benefit?

- What is the evidence supporting the claims of its effectiveness? Has a rigorous, scientific, evidence-based study been conducted and published in a credible cancer journal? Or is the information about its effectiveness only anecdotal, based on satisfied customers who have purchased the product?

- What are the risks of using this treatment? How safe is it? How was safety evaluated for this product/therapy?

- If someone is providing this therapy, what are his or her credentials to do so? Does he or she have a certification or a license? Some practitioners are licensed by state medical boards or accredited by professional organizations.

- Is the source of the therapy also the seller of the therapy? If so, they may have a vested interest in convincing people to purchase it. Sadly, some dishonest people will prey on individuals who are dealing with end-stage cancers.

There are two websites that provide tips to help you make decisions about the use of complementary and alternative medicine:

National Center for Complementary and Alternative Medicine of the National Institutes of Health at *www.nccam.nih.gov/health/decisions/index.htm*

Center for Food Safety and Applied Nutrition of the U.S. Food and Drug Administration at *www.cfan.fda.gov/~dms/ds-savvy.html.*

Before making any decisions to try something on your own, most specifically if it involves taking a product, discuss it with your doctor.

PART TEN

Other Common Questions

My family wants me to stop smoking, but I already have incurable cancer. Do I have to stop?

A friend of mine who has metastatic disease says that periodically she gets to stop treatment for a while. How does my oncologist decide if I can have a drug holiday? How long does it usually last?

I am tired of people telling me how good I look, which is commonly followed by, "Your cancer is gone, right?" How should I respond?

More . . .

86. My family wants me to stop smoking, but I already have incurable breast cancer. Do I have to stop?

You are not going to make your cancer worse by continuing to smoke, but there is some controversy on whether or not cigarette smoking makes the side effects of treatment worse. This is probably true of radiation therapy that involves any part of the upper gastrointestinal tract, especially the mouth and esophagus. Smoking is a well-known risk factor for pulmonary complications following general anesthesia for surgery. It may also increase your risk of developing blood clots or **pulmonary embolism** while on hormonal therapy. Although some oncologists believe that it increases the severity of mucositis (mouth sores and ulcers) from chemotherapy and other treatments, studies have shown that this effect is minimal, at most. Indeed, most studies have failed to show any dramatic increase in the side effects of most systemic therapy drugs in people who smoke, compared to those who do not.

Pulmonary embolism

Blockage of blood vessels in the lungs that interferes with breathing.

Stopping smoking is hard enough to do under the best of circumstances, and these are hardly the best of circumstances. On the other hand, some people getting systemic therapy do lose the taste for cigarettes. Others find that their diagnosis is just the motivation that they need to stop, especially when they see it as a way of setting a good example for their loved ones and friends. After all, they have everything to gain by kicking the habit. Even if your family members do not smoke, your smoking can jeopardize their health (*second-hand smoke*). If you are able to stop smoking, you will probably feel better, and that does go a long way to helping you handle the stresses of therapy and cancer. However, if your family wants you to stop, but you cannot, it probably is not worth the bad feelings that usually result from continuing to argue about it.

87. My doctor told me that I have a tumor in my liver. Is that the same as cancer?

Some doctors use words like *tumor, spot, neoplasm, lesion,* or *mass* to ease the emotional blow of the word *cancer.* However well meaning as it may be, this type of paternalism is not helpful. You need to know in clear terms your cancer has returned so that you can make appropriate decisions about how to deal with this reality. If your doctor refuses to speak with you honestly and directly, you need to find another doctor who will.

On the other hand, doctors often use words like *mass* or *spot* to describe an abnormality on a scan that he or she suspects could be cancer—but that could also be something else. In situations like this, your doctor will suggest a biopsy to confirm his suspicions. After a pathologist looks at this biopsy, your doctor will be able to tell you if it is cancer or not.

What is most important is that your doctor and you have good lines of communication—you both need to understand what is being said and make sure it matches what is being heard. So tell your doctor that you want the word *cancer* used if he or she is referring to cancer somewhere within your body. Also, it is common that an oncologist will give you information verbally and then ask you, "Do you understand?" Such a question only allows a "yes" or "no" response. If and when this occurs, tell the doctor, "Let me make sure I understand what you just told me. I will repeat it back in my own words to make sure I understood what

If your doctor refuses to speak with you honestly and directly, you need to find another doctor who will.

you said as you intended." Then tell the oncologist in your own words how you translated the information. Also, ask your nurse navigator to review the information with you again to ensure everyone understands what your current clinical situation is and what the next steps are going to be.

88. A friend of mine who has metastatic disease says that periodically she gets to stop treatment for a while. How does my oncologist decide if I can have a drug holiday? How long does it usually last?

The standard practice of most oncologists is to continue systemic therapy for as long as it is working or until you have unacceptable side effects. However, you and your oncologist may decide to stop chemotherapy for a while if you have metastatic disease that has been stable or in remission for some time. This may be particularly important to you if you are having considerable side effects from the treatment.

Overall survival

The percentage of people in a study who have survived for a certain period of time, usually reported as time since diagnosis or treatment. Often called the survival rate.

There are not a lot of studies to help you make this decision, but the limited information available suggests that while continuous therapy does not change **overall survival**, it does prolong the time that your cancer stays in remission (**progression-free survival**) when compared to shorter-course therapies. The downside of this is that continuous therapy is often associated with more side effects than shorter-course therapy. On the other hand, some people actually feel better getting therapy.

Progression-free survival

The length of time during and after treatment in which a patient is living with a disease that does not get worse. Progression-free survival may be used in a clinical study or trial to help find out how well a new treatment works.

Much of this depends on the particular systemic therapy program that you are getting. For example, it is unusual for someone to get more than 6 months of paclitaxel without having significant numbness and tingling in her fingers or toes (see Question 60). This dose-related peripheral neuropathy could cause severe pain and interfere with your ability to hold objects or walk. In fact, one study showed little difference in the time to breast cancer progression in a group of patients who got long-term, compared to short-term, paclitaxel.

If your cancer recurs but is **asymptomatic** (for example, your re-staging bone scan shows a few new small spots in the bones, but you have no pain), it may be quite reasonable for you to take a drug holiday for a few months. Knowing that your cancer is progressing, you and your oncologist can closely monitor the situation with scans, blood tests, and routine visits so that you can begin a new treatment regimen at the first sign of symptoms or change in the cancer's rate of growth.

Asymptomatic
Not manifesting any symptoms.

Emily's comments:

What a strange term—a drug holiday. But that is exactly what it is! I get to have a break for a while from taking medicines all the time. I feel that my body is getting a chance to recover from chemicals, and I know that I'm being monitored closely to ensure that it is safe for me to take a break from treatment for a while.

89. How do I know that I am getting the right treatments if my invasive lobular carcinoma isn't the more common form of breast cancer that would have been studied in clinical trials?

Invasive lobular carcinoma is not as common as invasive ductal carcinoma, but it's still the second most common form of breast cancer, accounting for approximately 15% of all breast cancers. And though it occurs less frequently, scientists and treating physicians still know quite a bit about it. It usually spreads to organs such as the stomach, colon, ovaries, and uterus and can also go to the more traditional metastatic sites including bone, liver, and lung. The majority of invasive lobular carcinomas are hormone receptor-positive, which makes hormonal therapies—and for those who are postmenopausal, CDK4/6 inhibitors—of great benefit to such patients. It commonly is HER2– as well. This type of breast cancer can grow more slowly than the more common invasive ductal carcinoma does. The same drug treatments are used based on the prognostic factors mentioned above, and the effectiveness of these therapies is determined in the same manner as for stage IV invasive ductal carcinoma.

90. I am tired of people telling me how good I look, which is commonly followed by, "Your cancer is gone, right?" How should I respond?

It is certainly understandable to be frustrated. People who know you very well and are in your inner circle are the ones you can talk to candidly and tell them how you are feeling. Those you see less frequently and don't feel as close to are usually the ones to make these kinds of comments. They may actually be feeling awkward seeing you, and for lack of a better comment to make they blurt out that you look good, which perhaps you do. They definitely don't feel comfortable talking about the "C-word," and therefore they are hoping that the cancer is gone, having basically no understanding of how stage IV breast cancer operates. You can thank the person for the compliment and respond with, "Thanks. I am feeling pretty good today compared to other days," or if you really feel crappy, you can say, "Thanks. I wish I felt as good as I apparently look." When it comes to the most significant statement, which is the one you feel angry about hearing, remember that most people don't live in the world you have become an expert in by having gotten stage IV breast cancer. So this is an opportunity for education. Tell the person that stage IV breast cancer is the type of breast cancer that cannot be cured, so you will always live with it and undergo various treatments for it. You also, of course, have the option of saying nothing and walking on. It is your choice.

Efforts are being made to educate the general public on your behalf about metastatic breast cancer. This is because research surveys of the general public conducted by Pfizer confirm that most people are very confused about this disease. The general public is so misinformed, in fact, that it is felt to be an imperative to educate consumers with the hope that fewer people will say the wrong thing to a patient or will assume the wrong things about how this breast cancer even happened. Your voice is being heard by the right people. They are advocating for you in a significant way. One of the outcomes of Pfizer's work in this space was the development of an educational tool called *The Story Half Told* (https://www.storyhalftold.com/). I had the privilege of helping to create this document accompanied by a PowerPoint presentation to bring to light the issues you are dealing with on a day-to-day basis, explaining just how uninformed the general public is about metastatic breast cancer, and even providing educational materials for employers so they can give better support for patients who are working during treatment or need time away for treatment and recovery. There you will find more information about the survey results as well as personal stories, perhaps similar to your own. This is a living, breathing document and has been shared with tens of thousands of oncology professionals as well as with stage IV breast cancer patients.

PART ELEVEN

End of Life, Treatment, Crossroads, Making Plans

How do I approach talking about end-of-life decisions with my family?

How and when will the doctor recommend that I stop treatment?

I feel very stressed about my medical situation and need time to clear my head and think about what I want to do. How can I get it?

More . . .

The goal of treatment of metastatic breast cancer is to sustain life while ensuring quality of life. There may be a point in time down the road when your doctor tells you news that you wish you didn't have to hear—that the treatments are no longer working and there aren't any other treatments to offer. This is the toughest discussion you and your doctor will ever have to undertake. It's shocking, depressing, overwhelming, frustrating, and not fair. But it happens.

Ideally, you and your doctor, as well as your family, have already had discussions about what lies ahead of you, including how to participate in the decisions about when YOU may want work toward preserving your quality of life without the involvement of potentially toxic treatments or even stop treatment altogether. You need to be the one in control, and for that, you must thoroughly understand your choices. Treatment for treatment's sake is bad care. Retrospective studies have proven that receiving treatment right up to the end of life shortens the patient's life. Some of the things that need to happen at this point in your journey are provided in this special chapter.

91. What is palliative care?

Palliative care is a philosophy of care that is intended to address your medical, physical, emotional, social, and spiritual needs. It is designed to help you have the best **quality of life** possible. Though originally created to be exclusively for patients at the end of life, this type of approach to treatment and care is now available for patients in active treatment, too.

The mission of palliative care is preserving or restoring your quality of life. Don't wait for your doctor to

Quality of life

The aspects of life that make it enjoyable and worth living. Cancer treatment balances the need to keep the body alive against whether the life is of acceptable quality.

make a referral. Request that a palliative care expert be added to your multidisciplinary team early on, even before you are having symptoms that warrant management. Palliative care really focuses on the whole patient in delivering patient-centered care. Palliative care specialists do their best to avoid using opioids for pain control, too.

Here are some questions for you to consider answering, even if you are not asked these questions by your oncologist or your palliative care doctor. The answers to these questions are a very good way of letting your treatment team know how you are doing emotionally. Your answers will change over time, so keep this list handy, and bring up these questions and provide your most current answers each time you are seen by your providers.

- How much do you know about your metastatic breast cancer?
- How much do you want to know about your metastatic breast cancer?
- What are you hoping for?
- What are you most worried about?
- What are three things that bring you joy?

92. What is an advance directive, and how can I make sure my wishes are known?

Advance directives are legal documents that allow you to state what type of medical care you want to receive if you become unable to make such decisions or speak on your own behalf in the future. Although the specific laws and terminology for advance directives may vary

Advance directive

A legal document that allows people to express their decisions regarding what they do and don't want to have done during their last weeks or months in case they become unable to communicate effectively.

from state to state, there are two basic types of advance directives: a living will and a healthcare proxy (discussed in detail in Question 93). Everyone, whether ill nor not, should have such documents in place. If you were not dealing with metastatic breast cancer right now, this would still be good advice to take. Think about it. Let's say you were in a serious auto accident, unconscious and unable to speak on your own behalf, and were to be taken to a trauma center by helicopter. The trauma team taking care of you needs to know what your expectations and desires are for treatment. Don't leave it to them to try to figure out. In the absence of such documents, the treatment team must take all measures to keep you alive, even if your brain isn't functioning well anymore. Is that what you would want? Now, in your current situation, you know you have stage IV breast cancer. If you slip into a coma, do you know what type of care you want to be receiving? Does your family know too? These wishes and expectations need to be documented. **Don't leave things to chance. This is also a way you still have control.**

> *The goal of treatment of metastatic breast cancer is to sustain life while ensuring quality of life.*

93. What is a living will? Is it the same as a healthcare proxy?

Living will

Outlines what care you want in the event you become unable to communicate because of coma or heavy sedation.

No. A **living will** is a special document in which you give specific instructions regarding your health care, particularly focusing on measures that relate to prolonging your life. A living will can describe which medical interventions you want to have done, as well as what you don't want performed, based on specific circumstances. For example, if you were unable to eat or drink anymore, would you want to have artificial nutrition through a feeding tube or receive nourishment with an IV? If your heart were to stop, would you want CPR performed? Would you want to be on a respirator?

It can be useful in making these types of decisions to differentiate between the types of medical problems that may occur. If the medical problems were treatable and reversible, you may want all measures taken to resuscitate you and support you. If the problem was one of progression of disease, and no treatments are available to help fight the cancer, you may not want to have extraordinary measures taken such as resuscitation to prolong your life. In that situation, some people want to be explicit about this and request to sign a "do not resuscitate" (DNR) order to ensure that none of these measures is taken. Making these types of decisions is very hard. Communicating them to your family members is important and an emotional challenge. It's important that your wishes are carried out, however, and this helps ensure that they are.

There are two limitations to a living will. Not all states recognize a living will. It is also impossible to imagine all the potential circumstances that might occur in the future regarding your health. There may be decisions that you simply haven't thought about yet or aren't ready to discuss and make decisions about.

These types of problems may be alleviated by designating a **healthcare proxy**. This is sometimes also referred to as a healthcare surrogate, a medical proxy, or a medical power of attorney. This person is authorized by you to make healthcare decisions on your behalf when you are not able to do so for yourself. He or she can decide which medical interventions will and won't be carried out—what will be performed and what will be

Healthcare proxy

A designated person authorized to make decisions regarding your medical treatment when you are unable to do so.

withheld. Though the details vary from one state to another, all states recognize the term *healthcare proxy*.

When choosing the person to serve in the important role as your healthcare proxy, be sure to choose someone you trust and who will make decisions based on what *you* want for *yourself*, not on what he or she wants for you or would want in your situation. This person can be a family member or a friend. Talk with the person about what you want to have done in the event such decisions are needed. It's especially important to discuss issues regarding sustaining life with artificial means so your wishes are clearly known and understood. You can change your proxy at any time, as well as change your decisions about what you need and want.

Make your family and friends aware of whom you have chosen as your healthcare proxy. It's important for everyone to support this individual in making decisions on your behalf. If you have completed a living will (and this is wise for everyone to do, even unrelated to their medical condition), share this with them as well. Inform all of your doctors and other members of your medical team what your wishes are, and give them copies of any advance directive documents you have signed. Each time you become an inpatient, the staff should automatically ask you if you have such documents and if you brought them with you so they can become part of your medical record.

If you were to be admitted to the hospital and didn't have one already prepared, you would be offered one to complete and sign, which will apply to your care during that specific hospital admission.

You can obtain state-specific advance directive forms from a lawyer, your doctor, or your local hospital. Forms for all 50 states, the District of Columbia, and Puerto Rico are also available online through the National Hospice and Palliative Care website (https://www.nhpco.org/patients-and-caregivers/advance-care-planning/).

94. How do I approach talking about end-of-life decisions with my family?

Having a discussion about what you would want if you were unable to make decisions for yourself can be difficult for most people, but it is wise to do. Even women not dealing with metastatic breast cancer should be taking such steps, since none of us knows when we may be in an auto accident or other medical crisis that warrants such decisions. You may want to discuss this with your loved ones but worry that it will upset them. Or you may worry that you will get upset while discussing this important issue. It is always better to discuss these things when you are feeling relatively well rather than waiting for a crisis to hit and having to discuss it at that time. This way, you can calmly think about it, express your wants and needs, and be clear about what you want to happen.

There are various ways you might begin this discussion. You might say something like "I want to be sure that if I were ever to become more ill than I am now, you would know what I want to have done." Sometimes family members don't agree with our decisions. This can make the discussion harder and, frankly, makes it even more important to be clear and have things documented. This is a good reason for an advance directive. Loved ones never want to picture you in a situation that warrants having to make decisions without your being able to speak for yourself. This is also an appropriate time to discuss what you want regarding a funeral. Again, this is a way to have control over a part of your life that carries significance to you. If you are not comfortable discussing that element of end of life, record on paper what you want done, providing as many details as possible. Families really struggle with having to decide on behalf of their loved one what they think and hope she would have wanted in these circumstances. Don't place that burden on them when it isn't necessary. And anyway, this is *your* life. You need and deserve to leave this world as you wish, with a viewing, funeral, cremation, and/or celebration of your life. Consider the same important steps when it comes to having a will describing the disposition of your estate. There may be specific things you want certain individuals to get. Unless these wishes are recorded, it may not happen. Again, it's a means for you to have control.

It is always better to discuss these things when you are feeling relatively well rather than waiting for a crisis to hit and have to discuss it at that time.

95. How and when will the doctor recommend that I stop treatment?

There may be a time when you and your oncologist have a serious discussion about how your treatment has been going. It may include a discussion about treatments that are no longer working and the lack of additional treatment options available. You may want to stay on a particular drug regimen, but your doctor may have determined that the treatment is no longer effective.

The doctor may tell you that the benefits from taking the treatment are too small in comparison to the side effects you are experiencing and will continue to experience, thus affecting the quality of your remaining life in a major way. The two of you may decide to change pathways from aggressively fighting the disease to beginning to prepare for the end of life. There is probably no harder decision than this one. In some cases, the patient makes the decision to end treatment herself. She may decide this based on how she feels and would rather focus on closure with family and friends and enjoy quality time with loved ones than continuing aggressive therapy.

There have been situations where no such discussion happens between the treating medical oncologist and the patient. This is truly unfortunate, because treating for the sake of giving some type of treatment isn't factoring in the patient's personal goals and quality-of-life needs. It's important to weigh the goals of treatment against the goals the patient has for her life. Some patients expect the doctor to bring up the issue of stopping treatment, and some doctors delay the discussion, anticipating the patient will initiate it. The result is that the patient doesn't always have the opportunity to prepare for the end of life as she had anticipated, leaving family members to make decisions that they are not prepared for. There are no rules about this and no specific guidelines to be followed; however, it is considered "bad care" if a patient is still receiving drug treatments within 3 weeks of her death. Some people decide to continue treatment until the last possible moment, and others choose to stop earlier. Remember, the decision to stop treatment can be reversed if you wish. Talking with your family and doctors about it can help you decide what is realistic. It is appropriate to be optimistic about getting this disease under control. That is the goal, after all. If there is a time that realism takes over optimism, then making the decision can be done with you in a thoughtful way with your oncologist's help and family's support.

It is very unfortunate to be working with a medical oncologist who has difficulty having such discussions and will continue treatment for as long as possible, even if it is not helping you anymore. The oncologist may be waiting for you to be too ill from its side effects and having with worsening symptoms caused by the further spreading of the cancer. This is why it is important for *you* to make decisions for yourself how long you want to continue treatment. As each treatment over time stops working and you are switched to another therapy, usually the length of time it helps you diminishes while the side effects increase. Remember, quality of life should be the goal rather than just looking at quantity of life. If you are only existing and not enjoying your life, then it's time to have a serious discussion—first with yourself, then with your family, then with your medical oncologist. It has been clinically proven that metastatic breast cancer patients who discontinue aggressive treatments sooner actually live longer with a better quality of life. Don't feel obligated to continue treatments to please your doctor or your family, either. This is your life; no one else's. You are not surrendering to the disease; instead, you are regaining control of how you want to spend the remainder of your life—at home, with hospice care, and friends and family around you. You may even be able to squeeze in a few more things from your bucket list that you didn't anticipate would be possible.

Hospice

An organization that provides programs and services designed to help alleviate the physical and psychosocial suffering associated with progressive, incurable illness.

96. My doctor says that it's time to get hospice involved and stop my treatment. What is hospice, and what can I expect them to help me with?

Hospice tries to help the patient and her close family members prepare for the end of life. Hospice's mission is to improve the quality of life for individuals with health problems that are considered fatal. Hospice helps with (1) pain relief and other medical supportive care; (2) emotional and spiritual support for you and your family; and (3) help with daily tasks such as bathing, dressing, and other activities of daily living. They can also be instrumental in helping reduce financial expenses associated with end-of-life cancer care by obtaining prescription medicines at cost; arranging for a hospital bed, commode, wheelchair, and other medical equipment that may be needed at home; as well as providing hospice nurses and home health aides to come to you on a routine basis. For patients who prefer not to be in the home and would rather be in a hospice facility, your doctor will arrange for admission to such a place that will be as close to your home as possible to make it convenient for your family and friends to see and spend time with you. Hospice facilities have an open-door policy of permitting visitors 24/7. Hospice also provides spiritual counselors, depending on your religious faith and personal desires and needs. Many insurance companies cover hospice care. If you are over 65, you probably qualify for the Medicare hospice benefit. You may want to check with your insurance company if they have a relationship with specific hospice care units in your geographic region. For more information on hospice, call the Hospice Foundation of America at 800-854-3402.

Hospice and palliative care work together now, still striving to get symptom management including pain into control for you. Today, the average number of days that someone receives hospice care is just 5 days. It is designed to be for 6 months, however. Why the wide gap? In part, this is due to some doctors being hesitant to mention it, wanting to continue treatments for as long as possible, even when it is not in the patient's best interest. Remember, how long you get treatment is your decision, no one else's. Always weigh the risks and benefits of each line of therapy as they are presented to you. Some people may actually say to you, "Why have you decided to not fight anymore?" Tell them you have chosen to regain control over your life. Remember, we knew from the beginning that cure wasn't possible, so you were never fighting for a cure. You have been getting treatment to control the disease while hopefully maintaining quality of life, as you define it. Family members can also be upset that you have chosen to stop treatment. Remind them that this needs to be your decision. Do not be swayed by someone saying, "Do one more treatment for me." Such arguments are unfair to you. It is a strange phenomenon, but as long as a loved one is still breathing, family members seem okay with the situation, forgetting that their loved one is no longer thriving or truly living out the remainder of her life as she wants to. And when the time comes to take this stand, tell your loved ones that they need to love you enough to let you make your own decisions at this important juncture in your journey.

Hospice's mission is to improve the quality of life for individuals with health problems that they are no longer able to treat and are considered fatal.

Tia's comments:

I worry about how my kids will cope with my dying. Though I admit I'm scared, I know it scares them even more. It's time I met with my hospice chaplain to discuss this and get some insight as to what they may be thinking and how I can get closure as well as feel that they will be okay after I'm gone. It's been wonderful how comfortable I have felt talking with the hospice staff. They are obviously much more experienced than I am in these things and I appreciate having them here for support and as a sounding board.

97. I want my children to remember me. I also want to help them cope with my having to leave them. What can you suggest to help us with both?

For children who are young, it's important for them to understand that nothing they have done has caused this to happen. Young children sometimes think they have wished this on their mother. They may have thought something like, "Mommy wouldn't let me play at Joey's house. I wish she were dead. She is mean to me." They literally think that they have caused your illness and death to happen. Make it clear that nothing they have done has caused the cancer. Let them know that cancer is not contagious.

Teens and preteens can feel a real sense of anxiety and distress. Older children who are out on their own, perhaps with their own families, will surely feel pain and loss but are better equipped emotionally to deal with this than young people are. For any children still living at home and dependent on you, emphasize to them that they will be taken care of, no matter what happens.

For children under the age of 25, consider getting cards for each of them—cards for each birthday up through age 21, graduation from high school, from college; cards for significant holidays you celebrate together, such as Easter, Christmas, Rosh Hashanah; cards for when they marry and when they have their first child. Write one or two sentences on each card that is specific for that date. What do you want to tell your child on this day (for example, when she turns sweet 16)? You can still be "right there," instilling your values in your children by doing this, and they will greatly value these cards as they grow up. In order to do this, you will need to recruit the assistance of the card store manager because some cards are seasonal (and stored in the back room). Explain your situation, or if you are not able to go yourself, ask a family member to go on your behalf. Put the name of the child and the date/milestone event it is to be opened on the outside of the envelope and have them stored in a safety deposit box rather than in your or someone's home. These cards are not replaceable later; if there were to be a flood or fire, they would be lost. It's worth the money each year to rent a safety deposit box at a local bank. Select a family member to be responsible for their timely distribution. Your children will sense your presence at the time of each milestone in their lives.

An additional idea for daughters, for whom the loss of their role-model parent may be particularly acute, is to create a charm bracelet for her that contains milestones she has already reached or favorite places the two of you have enjoyed together. Then purchase additional charms to be added later. A graduation cap for graduation from high school, a Sweet 16 charm for her 16th birthday, or wedding bells for when she marries.

Be sure your wishes are known regarding who you want to receive special mementos you own, such as specific pieces of jewelry. Don't leave this for your family to decipher alone, if it can be avoided. What you want done with these things is important for them to know. Your heart will tell you what to do. They certainly know it is not your choice to succumb to this disease. Fate has dealt you a hand that wasn't your doing or theirs.

Johns Hopkins holds metastatic breast cancer retreats semiannually for patients like you who are dealing with stage IV breast cancer. One is for couples, so the patient brings her spouse/partner; the other one is for women not in a relationship, so they bring a female caregiver. These programs, which last 3 days and 2 nights, are free to attend, funded by philanthropy and foundation grants. Attendees do need to provide their own transportation. I developed and implemented these retreats in 2006. It is a wonderful way to get to meet others like you for networking, have your loved one accompanying you do the same with other family caregivers, learn new coping skills, stress management exercises, talk about some of the tough decisions you are in need of making or soon perhaps will be, have respite time, reduce anxiety, get a massage by a certified oncology massage therapist, participate in seated gentle yoga, and even participate in activities that will bring genuine belly laughs. I have been helping other breast centers replicate these retreats for their stage IV breast cancer patients, too. The Hopkins retreats are not restricted to Hopkins patients either, so consider inquiring when our retreats are next happening and get registered. These retreats are held at a Spiritual Center outside of Baltimore, with 362 acres of serenity, private rooms, private baths, and excellent menu options. The hardest part is always having to go home and leave the new friends you have made. Each group that attends the retreats creates a closed Facebook page to continue to remain connected for a long time to come. For information, email me at shockli@jhmi.edu. I can also speak with your nurse navigator or other support staff on your multidisciplinary team to see if they want to get a copy of a detailed program planning guide how to launch these retreats for you and other patients cared for at your facility where you are getting your treatment. I also may know some excellent funding sources to make it even easier for your breast center to replicate this type of program.

Lauren's comments:

Selecting cards for my children to have as they grow up without me was very hard at first. Then, as I began to write in each one what my wishes were for them on that significant day in their lives, I felt better. This will be one of the ways I feel I will still be here for my children, instilling my value system in them and telling them my hopes and dreams for their futures.

98. I feel very stressed about my medical situation and need time to clear my head and think about what I want to do. How can I get it?

Sometimes it is advisable to request to meet with a social worker or counselor for assistance. If you are involved with hospice, let the hospice staff taking care of you know you are distressed. This is not the time to hide it or try to see if the feelings of anxiety will pass. You are in an extraordinary situation, and it is perfectly normal to feel upset.

You need to find ways to relieve your stress and reduce your fears. Some ways to do this are:

- Take a walk or exercise. Nothing strenuous, but power walking or treadmill walking are good options.
- Keep a journal of your thoughts and feelings. Writing them down is very therapeutic.
- Meditation, prayer, or performing relaxation exercises that include deep breathing are helpful.
- Talk with someone such as a close friend, clergy, or counselor about your fears and anxieties.

- Consider joining a support group. Some breast centers offer special support groups for women dealing with metastatic disease.
- Join an online support group.
- Listen to soothing music or a CD of sounds like the ocean or birds chirping.
- Create a work of art that displays your feelings and thoughts. There are some breast centers that offer art therapy. You don't have to be an artist to do this. A simple drawing or creation from clay can be done. It's your work of art. You don't have to share it with anyone unless you choose to do so.
- Do yoga.
- Spend time with close friends with whom you can be yourself. Talk, read from a joke book, watch a funny movie, listen to music together, eat dessert. All of this is good for you, good for them, and good for the soul.

Return to the list of questions discussed earlier that you need to keep in the forefront and answer for yourself, for your family, and for your treatment team.

- How much do you know about your breast cancer?
- How much do you want to know about your breast cancer?
- What are you hoping for?
- What are you most worried about?
- What are three things that bring you joy?

Right now, focus on the last question: What are three things that bring you joy? Don't postpone joy, ever. Do make plans for doing various simple activities that you love or know you will enjoy. Don't get caught up in the question of, "What if I don't feel well enough to go next

Wednesday with my girlfriends to the movies?" Go ahead and make the plans. If you feel well enough to go, then great! If you don't, then have them come over to you on a different day and watch a chick flick at home.

You will also find that simple things become noticeable and part of your joy each day. Seeing a robin sitting on her nest. Watching toddlers playing and laughing in your neighbor's yard. Music may hold greater importance to you now. Ask a friend to create a DVD of specific songs you love so you can play it whenever you like. Skype or FaceTime with a grandchild and learn what is happening in their world. All of these things that seemed mundane probably in the past now hold a different meaning for you.

99. How do I decide what is the best way to be spending my time if the doctor tells me that my time is limited? Do I still work as much as I can? Do I take a trip? How do I make these decisions?

Often, as we are going through our daily routine, we don't realize how precious time is. It's not until we learn that we have a limited amount of it that we recognize just how precious it is. Sit and talk with your loved ones about these decisions. You have the right to spend it as you want and not to feel pressure to maintain your old routine, especially if you were overloaded with responsibilities. If you enjoy doing these things, then do them. If you don't, then discuss with your family how you would prefer to spend your time. It may be seeing grandchildren more often. You may wish to take a trip. If that isn't realistic, based on how you are feeling, then get a movie (IMAX, if available) of the place you long to see and take a virtual trip there. This is a time to express your thoughts and feelings more openly and to let people know what your concerns, wishes, and hopes are, especially for those you will leave behind. For many this may be a spiritual time. For others it may be a time to spend resting with briefer visits by family and friends. Keep a journal, too, of the things that are bringing you joy, big and small.

I gave one key piece of advice earlier, and I'll emphasize it again here: **DON'T POSTPONE JOY**. There is a tendency to want to delay a vacation until later, but when later comes, you may be too ill to enjoy it. Do things now while you are able. Avoid regrets later. We cannot rewind the clock.

100. I have heard that the best way to prepare for the end of life is to reflect back over my life. What would I be trying to accomplish by doing this? Someone told me it is a way to help ensure I experience a good death. I don't understand what I am to get out of such an exercise. It sounds scary.

No one likes to talk about death in general. But it will happen to everyone. You are in a unique situation of having a better idea of how soon it may happen to you, however. This provides an unusual opportunity—you can help orchestrate for yourself a good, peaceful death. Here are the key elements that are required for you to experience a good and peaceful death. It is never too soon to read them over and begin the necessary steps to ensure yours are all fulfilled:

1. Knowing you had a purpose for living and it was valued by at least one other person

2. Leaving a legacy, unrelated to leaving money for some purpose. (This could be a philosophy you have about living life to the fullest. It might be teaching others to be kind. Being an extraordinary cook and leaving recipes for your daughters to continue your way of preparing special holiday meals. One of your legacies might be to have participated in a clinical trial. And yes, it could be leaving a donation for something that is important to you. The message here is that it doesn't have to be about money.)

3. Having all of your legal and financial affairs in order. Your doctor may have said to you, "I recommend that you get your affairs in order," but that doesn't mean you know what to do. There are great resources to guide you through this that are online as well as on various websites. If you attend a retreat as mentioned earlier, you will receive an end-of-life planning guide for you and your family. You should meet with a lawyer to ensure your will is up-to-date and meet with an accountant to ensure your financial affairs are squared away. Though it may not feel good to do these things, it is the smart thing to do, because, again, it gives you control. People who die without these things in order leave their family with a mess to address, and Uncle Sam will relieve them of more money than you intended the government to get. Everyone should have their affairs in order—not just you. Your spouse could be in a fatal car crash even before

you are gone. Are his affairs in order? It is the right thing to do, a loving thing to do, and you get to determine the disposition of everything that is yours.

4. Leaving no financial debt associated with your cancer care for your family to have to pay. This is really important to most individuals. Even though family members may have said that they are happy to cover whatever expenses that may be incurred that you are not able to cover for yourself, it can be a large sum of money. So when discussing treatment options with your treatment team, meet with a financial coun- selor or financial navigator to find out what out-of-pocket expenses you are going to incur by having this treatment. It will become one of the decision makers you use to do a specific treatment or not to do that treatment now. Also inquire of your treatment team whether there are discounted drug programs offered by the pharmaceutical companies that manufacture the drug(s) too.

5. Giving forgiveness and receiving forgiveness. This cannot be accomplished in just a weekend. It requires thought. And it doesn't mean you forgive everyone you feel has done you wrong. But you do have to think about it and make de- cisions about it. Are there also people you want to receive forgiveness from? Consider writing a letter or calling them on the phone. If comfort- able, invite them over for a talk. Clearing the air is very freeing.

6. Being pain free. Remember, that is what pallia- tive care can help accomplish for you. There is no reason to be suffering in pain.

7. Dying with dignity in the environment of your own choosing. When asked, most patients say they want to be home with hospice care. However, only 23% of metastatic cancer patients get asked, and 24% of metastatic (solid organ) cancer patients actually die in an ICU on a respirator—which means there was no discussion about when to stop treatment or how to choose a pathway of control by stopping treatment and enrolling in hospice.

8. Feeling confident you will be spoken of fondly after you are gone. This is really important. Sometimes it comes up in discussion if the patient wants to plan her own funeral or celebration of life ceremony. Even what someone wears while lying in a casket can hold great meaning to them and to those visiting them and their family at a funeral home.

9. Feeling connected spiritually to a higher power. For some patients, there is a connection early on because of their belief system before they were diagnosed. For others, they may be angry with God and not feel a connection at all. Most, however, do feel a spiritual connection, even if it isn't until close to their own passing. This is personal and must be approached personally and privately. Talking with a hospice chaplain has been helpful for many patients as well as for their families. It's something to consider.

With these elements fulfilled, and receiving effective hospice and palliative care, a smoother journey to the end of life can and will be possible.

The verse below provides comfort to many family members, as well as to friends and even to patients who have some type of serious, life-limiting illness.

I stand at the shore—a ship spread her white sails to the morning breeze and starts for the blue ocean. She is an object of beauty and strength as I watch her like a speck of white cloud just where the sea and sky come down to mingle with each other. Then someone at my side says, "There, she is gone!"

Gone? Gone where? Gone from my sight, that is all. She is just as large in mast and hull and spar as she was when she left my side . . . and just as able to bear her load of living freight to the place of her destination.

Her diminished size is in me, not in her; and just at the moment that someone at my side says, "There, she is gone," there are other eyes watching and other voices ready to take up the glad shout, "Here she comes!"

—Henry Van Dyke

PART TWELVE

Breast Cancer Drug Therapy Information

Table 1 Drugs Used in the Treatment of Breast Cancer

Drug Name Generic (Brand), Maker	Actions/Common Side Effects*
CHEMOTHERAPY	**The treatment of cancer using specific chemical agents or drugs that are selectively destructive to malignant cells and tissues.**
ALKYLATING AGENTS	Alkylating agents are a group of chemotherapy drugs that target the DNA of cancer cells to prevent the cells from growing or reproducing. Alkylating agents attack cancer cells in all phases and disrupt their growth. These cells are then destroyed.
Cyclophosphamide (*Cytoxan*) Bristol-Myers Squibb	Cyclophosphamide (Cytoxan) is a chemotherapy drug commonly used to treat breast cancer and other cancers. Cyclophosphamide first disrupts cancer cells, then destroys them. Cyclophosphamide is taken in tablets by mouth or intravenously (through the vein) over 30–60 minutes. Side effects may include decrease in blood cell counts with increased risk of infection; nausea, vomiting, diarrhea, and abdominal pain; decreased appetite; hair loss (reversible); bladder damage; fertility impairment; lung and hearing damage (with high doses); sores in mouth or on lips; and stopping of menstrual periods. Less common side effects: decreased platelet count (mild) with increased risk of bleeding, blood in urine, darkening of nail beds, acne, fatigue, fetal changes if patient becomes pregnant when taking

(Continues)

Table 1 Drugs Used in the Treatment of Breast Cancer (*Continued*)

Drug Name Generic (Brand), Maker	Actions/Common Side Effects*
	cyclophosphamide. At high doses, can cause heart problems. Urinary system problems and some secondary cancers have been reported.
ANTHRACYCLINE ANTIBIOTICS	**Anthracyclines work by deforming the DNA structure of cancer cells and terminating their biological function. They disrupt the growth of cancer cells, which are then destroyed.**
Doxorubicin (*Adriamycin*) Pfizer	Doxorubicin (Adriamycin) is a type of antibiotic used specifically in the treatment of cancer. It interferes with the multiplication of cancer cells and slows or stops their growth and spread in the body. Side effects may include decreased white blood cell count with increased risk of infection, decreased platelet count with increased risk of bleeding, loss of appetite, darkening of nail beds and skin creases of hands, hair loss, damage to the skin if drug gets outside the veins, nausea, and vomiting. Less common side effects: sores in mouth or on lips, radiation recall skin changes, fetal abnormalities if taken while pregnant or if patient becomes pregnant while on this drug. Patients should be tested for heart problems before beginning doxorubicin and should be continuously monitored for developing problems during treatment.
Epirubicin (*Ellence*) Pfizer	Epirubicin (Ellence) was approved by the FDA in 1999 to treat early-stage breast cancer after breast surgery (lumpectomy or mastectomy) in patients whose cancer has spread to the lymph nodes. Epirubicin helps reduce the likelihood that breast cancer will return and improves a patient's chances of survival. Epirubicin is given intravenously (through the vein) in combination with two other chemotherapy drugs, cyclophosphamide and fluorouracil. Side effects may include nausea, vomiting, diarrhea, inflammation of the mouth, hair loss, damage to the skin if drug gets out of the veins, and reduction in white blood cells. Less common side effects: There is a risk of irreversible damage to the heart muscle associated with the drug. For women

Drug Name Generic (Brand), Maker	Actions/Common Side Effects*
	who receive epirubicin as adjuvant therapy, there is a slightly increased risk of treatment-related leukemia. Epirubicin may cause harm to the fetus if taken while pregnant.
ANTIMETABOLITES	**Antimetabolites prevent cells from making DNA and RNA by interfering with the synthesis of nucleic acids, thus disrupting the growth of cancer cells.**
5-Fluorouracil (*5-FU, Adrucil, Fluorouracil*) multiple makers	5-Fluorouracil is a drug that kills cancer cells by stopping their growth. It can also make it hard for cancer cells to fix damage. Side effects may include decreased white blood cell count with increased risk of infection; decreased platelet count with increased risk of bleeding; drowsiness or confusion; darkening of skin and nail beds; dry, flaky skin; nausea; vomiting; sores in mouth or on lips; thinning hair; diarrhea; brittle nails; and increased sensitivity to sun. Less common side effects: darkening and stiffening of vein used for giving the drug, decreased appetite, headache, weakness, and muscle aches. Cardiac symptoms are rare but are most likely in patients with ischemic heart disease.
Capecitabine (*Xeloda*) Roche	Capecitabine (Xeloda) is approved as a treatment for advanced breast cancer. Capecitabine works by converting to 5-fluorouracil (5-FU) in the body. It is used for cancers resistant to both paclitaxel and anthracyclines. Side effects may include diarrhea, nausea, vomiting, loss of appetite or decreased appetite and dehydration, sores in mouth or on lips, numbness, tingling, itching of hands and/or feet, skin redness, rash, dryness, decreased white blood cell count with increased risk of infection, decreased platelet count with increased risk of bleeding, decreased red blood cell count with increased risk of fatigue, and irritation of the skin. Less common side effects: abdominal pain, constipation, heartburn after eating, fever, sensation of pins and needles in hands and/or feet, headache, dizziness, difficulty falling asleep, eye irritation, and increased value of blood tests for liver function.

(Continues)

Table 1 Drugs Used in the Treatment of Breast Cancer (*Continued*)

Drug Name Generic (Brand), Maker	Actions/Common Side Effects*
Gemcitabine (*Gemzar*) Lilly Oncology	Gemcitabine (Gemzar) is approved as a treatment for advanced breast cancer in combination with paclitaxel. Side effects may include decreased blood counts with increased risk of infection, bleeding, and fatigue; nausea; vomiting; and skin rash. Less common side effects: fever, flu-like symptoms, swelling (edema), hair loss, and itching.
Ixabepilone (*Ixempra*) Bristol-Myers Squibb	Ixabepilone is approved for the treatment of aggressive metastatic or locally advanced breast cancer no longer responding to currently available chemotherapies. Ixabepilone is administered through injection, in combination with capecitabine for the treatment of advanced breast cancer in patients after failure of an anthracycline and a taxane.
Methotrexate (*MTX, Amethopterin, Folex, Mexate*) multiple makers	Methotrexate prevents cells from making DNA and RNA by interfering with the synthesis of nucleic acids, thus stopping the growth of cancer cells. Side effects may include nausea (high dose), vomiting (high dose), sores in mouth or on lips, diarrhea, increased risk of sunburn, radiation recall skin changes, and loss of appetite. Less common side effects: decreased white blood cell count with increased risk of infection, decreased platelet count with increased risk of bleeding, and kidney damage (high dose). Liver, lung, and nerve damage are sometimes seen with methotrexate use, but the adjuvant drug, leucovorin, offsets the worst side effects.

ANTINEOPLASTIC AGENT

Thiotepa (*Thioplex*) Various manufacturers	Thiotepa is an older cytotoxic agent chemically and pharmacologically similar to nitrogen mustard. It was widely used to treat breast cancers in the past, though at present it has been surpassed by other, more targeted therapeutic agents. It causes a wide range of side effects and is now rarely used in breast cancer treatment.

Drug Name Generic (Brand), Maker	Actions/Common Side Effects*
MICROTUBULE INHIBITOR	
Eribulin mesylate (*Halaven*) Eisai Co., Ltd.	Eribulin (Halaven) is a synthetic form of a chemo-therapeutically active compound derived from the sea sponge *Halichondria okadai*. This injectable therapy is a microtubule inhibitor, believed to work by inhibiting cancer cell growth. Before receiving eribulin, patients should have received prior anthracycline- and taxane-based chemotherapy for early- or late-stage breast cancer. It is an FDA-approved therapy used to treat late-stage, aggressive breast cancer that is no longer responding to other chemotherapy agents.
	Eribulin's safety and effectiveness were established in a single study in 762 women with metastatic breast cancer who had received at least two prior chemo-therapy regimens for late-stage disease. Patients were randomly assigned to receive treatment with either eribulin or a different single-agent therapy chosen by their oncologist.
	The study was designed to measure the length of time from when this treatment started until a patient's death (overall survival). The median overall survival for patients receiving eribulin was 13.1 months compared with 10.6 months for those who received a single-agent therapy.
	The most common side effects reported by women treated with eribulin include a decrease in infection-fighting white blood cells (neutropenia), anemia, a decrease in the number of white blood cells (leukope-nia), hair loss (alopecia), fatigue, nausea, weakness (asthenia), nerve damage (peripheral neuropathy), and constipation.
TAXANES	**Taxanes are powerful drugs that can stop cancer cells from repairing themselves and making new cells. Often used for treatment of cancers that have not responded to or have recurred after anthracycline therapy.**

(Continues)

Table 1 Drugs Used in the Treatment of Breast Cancer (*Continued*)

Drug Name Generic (Brand), Maker	Actions/Common Side Effects*
Docetaxel (*Taxotere*) Sanofi-Aventis	The FDA has approved docetaxel to be used as a single agent over a wide range of doses for the treatment of locally advanced or metastatic breast cancer in patients who have received prior chemotherapy. Docetaxel is also approved in combination with doxorubicin and cyclophosphamide for the adjuvant treatment of patients with operable, node-positive breast cancer. Docetaxel inhibits the division of breast cancer cells by acting on the cell's internal skeleton. Side effects may include decreased white blood cell count with increased risk of infection, decreased platelet count with increased risk of bleeding, hair thinning or loss, diarrhea, loss of appetite, nausea, vomiting, rash, and numbness and tingling in hands and/or feet related to peripheral nerve irritation or damage. Less common side effects: sores in mouth or on lips, swelling of ankles or hands, increased weight due to fluid retention, fatigue, muscle aches, loss of nails, and redness or irritation of the palms of hands or soles of feet.
Paclitaxel (*Taxol*) Bristol-Myers Squibb	Paclitaxel (Taxol) was first approved by the FDA in 1992 to treat advanced (metastatic) breast cancer. In 1999, the FDA also approved paclitaxel to treat early-stage breast cancer in patients who have already received chemotherapy with the drug doxorubicin. Paclitaxel is called a mitotic inhibitor because of its interference with cells during mitosis (cell division). Side effects may include decreased white blood cell count with increased risk of infection, fatigue, numbness and tingling in hands and/or feet related to peripheral nerve irritation or damage, muscle and bone aches for 3 days, hair loss, nausea, vomiting, mild diarrhea, and mild stomatitis. Less common side effects: allergic reaction: skin rash, flushing, increased heart rate, wheezing, and swelling of the face. Transient heart problems such as bradycardia occur in 30% or less of patients and are usually not severe.

Drug Name Generic (Brand), Maker	Actions/Common Side Effects*
VINCA ALKALOIDS	**A medication in a class of anticancer drugs that inhibits cancer cell growth by stopping cell division (mitosis).**
Vinblastine (generic) Fresenius Kabi	Vinblastine is the salt of an alkaloid extracted from *Vinca rosea* Linn., a common flowering herb known as the periwinkle. This agent causes cancer cells to be arrested in metaphase. It is not used as a first-line treatment for breast cancer but may be used in breast cancer that does not respond to hormonal or targeted therapy (e.g., triple-negative cancers). It causes a number of significant side effects, including low white and red blood cell counts, hair loss, gastrointestinal symptoms, high blood pressure, and numbness or tingling in the extremities.
Vinorelbine (*Navelbine*) GlaxoSmithKline	Vinorelbine (Navelbine) is used to treat metastatic breast cancer. Side effects may include decreased blood counts with increased risk of infection and damage to the skin if drug gets outside the vein. Less common side effects: numbness and tingling of hands and feet, nausea, and vomiting.
TARGETED THERAPY	**Targeted therapy is a general term that refers to a medication or drug that targets a specific pathway in the growth and development of a tumor. By attacking or blocking these important targets, the therapy helps to fight the tumor itself.**
MONOCLONAL ANTIBODIES (BIOLOGIC AGENTS)	**Monoclonal antibodies work by attaching to a specific protein on cancer cells like a key in a lock, potentially creating an immune response that can help kill the cancer cells. Biologic agents are drugs produced from living organisms or cells. Some targeted therapies are biologics.**
Atezolizumab (*Tencentriq*) Genentech	Atezolizumab is a programmed cell death ligand 1 (PD-L1)–blocking antibody. It is prescribed for the treatment of adult patients with unresectable locally advanced or metastatic triple-negative breast cancer (TNBC) whose tumors express PD-L1 (PD-L1–stained tumor-infiltrating immune cells [IC] of any intensity covering $\geq$1% of the tumor area), as determined by

(Continues)

Table 1 Drugs Used in the Treatment of Breast Cancer (*Continued*)

Drug Name Generic (Brand), Maker	Actions/Common Side Effects*
	an FDA-approved test. Key side effects include a number of immune-mediated inflammatory conditions, including pneumonitis, hepatitis, colitis, endocrinopathies, and uveitis, among others.
Lapatinib (*Tykerb*) Novartis	Lapatinib (Tykerb) is used to treat advanced or metastatic breast cancer that overexpresses the HER2 protein. It is usually given in combination with capecitabine, after prior therapies. Possible serious side effects include development of lung problems and certain heart problems, including congestive heart failure. More common side effects may include rash, skin blistering, diarrhea, indigestion, nausea, vomiting, liver problems, anemia, bleeding or bruising, backache, arm or leg pain, problems sleeping, and shortness of breath.
Pertuzumab (*Perjeta*) Genentech	Pertuzumab inhibits intracellular signaling through two major signaling pathways, mitogen-activated protein (MAP) kinase, and phosphoinositide 3-kinase (PI3K). Inhibition of these signaling pathways can result in cell growth arrest and apoptosis, respectively. It is used to treat HER2+ metastatic breast cancer. Pertuzumab's side effects include a black-box warning of left ventricular dysfunction requiring monitoring of cardiac function before and during treatment.
Trastuzumab (*Herceptin*) Genentech	Trastuzumab (Herceptin) is an FDA-approved therapeutic for HER2 protein–overexpressing metastatic breast cancer. Trastuzumab is a therapy for women with metastatic breast cancer whose tumors have too much HER2 protein. For patients with this disease, trastuzumab is approved for first-line use in combination with paclitaxel and as a single agent for those who have received one or more chemotherapy regimens. Possible serious side effects include development of certain heart problems, including congestive heart failure; severe allergic reactions; infusion reactions; lung problems; blood clots; or a reduction in white blood cells. Other side effects may include fatigue, infections, low white or red blood cell counts, trouble breathing, rash/skin blistering, constipation, headache, and muscle pain.

Drug Name Generic (Brand), Maker	Actions/Common Side Effects*
ADJUVANT THERAPY	**A variety of drugs that complement the chemo-therapy regimen.**
Folinic acid (*Leucovorin*) Pfizer	Leucovorin is a form of vitamin used to offset the side effects of methotrexate and/or enhance the action of 5-FU. Leucovorin has few side effects itself, but its use with 5-FU can sometimes exacerbate the side effects of that drug.
Pamidronate (*Aredia*) Novartis Zoledronic acid (*Zometa*) Novartis	Both pamidronate and zoledronic acid are used to alleviate hypercalcemia; zoledronic acid is a newer, more powerful agent. They also work to reduce the severity of osteoporosis. Both drugs have similar side effects, which may include fever lasting for a short time (24–48 hours after infusion), pain at place of injection, and irritation of the vein used for giving the drug. Less common side effects: nausea, constipation, anemia, and decreased appetite. Renal function should be monitored with use of zoledronic acid. Zoledronic acid can cause bone damage (osteonecrosis) in the jaw.
ANTIEMETIC MEDICATIONS	**Medications used to treat nausea and vomiting related to chemotherapy.**
Serotonin receptor antagonists (5-HT3 RAs) • Granisetron hydrochloride (*Kytril*) Roche • Dolasetron mesylate (*Anzemet*) Sanofi • Ondansetron hydrochloride (*Zofran*) GlaxoSmithKline • Palonesetron (*Aloxi*) Eisai Co., Ltd.	Serotonin receptor antagonists (5-HT3 Ras) are used to prevent nausea and vomiting.
Substance P/neurokinin (NK1) receptor antagonist • Aprepitant (*Emend*) Merck	Substance P/NK$_1$ receptor antagonists block nausea and vomiting pathways. They are given with a serotonin antagonist and dexamethasone to prevent nausea and vomiting.

(Continues)

Table 1 Drugs Used in the Treatment of Breast Cancer (*Continued*)

Drug Name Generic (Brand), Maker	Actions/Common Side Effects*
KINASE INHIBITORS	**Medications used to improve the ability of standard chemotherapy drugs to kill cancer cells.**
Abemaciclib (*Verzenio*) Eli Lilly & Co.	Abemaciclib inhibits cyclin-dependent kinases 4 and 6 (CDK4 and CDK6). It is used in treatment of HR+, HER2− metastatic breast cancer in conjunction with an aromatase inhibitor or fulvestrant. It may also be used by itself in HR+/HER2− metastatic breast cancer in patients who show progression of disease after hormonal therapy and chemotherapy. Side effects include diarrhea, low white blood cell count, venous thromboembolism, and interstitial lung disease/pneumonitis.
Alpelisib (*Piqray*) Novartis	Alpelisib inhibits phosphatidylinositol-3-kinase (PI3K) and is used in combination with fulvestrant to treat HR+/HER2− advanced or metastatic breast cancer that is PIK3CA-mutated, as detected by an FDA-approved test, following progression on or after an endocrine-based regimen. Side effects include elevated blood sugar, rash, and diarrhea.
Everolimus (*Afinitor, Afinitor Disperz*) Novartis	Everolimus inhibits mTOR, a serine-threonine kinase. It is used in combination with exemestane for treating postmenopausal women with HR+/HER2− breast cancer after unsuccessful treatment with letrozole or anastrozole. Everolimus has immunosuppressant properties that leave the patient vulnerable to infections, including opportunistic pathogens and invasive fungal infections. The rate of adverse reactions is high (>10%) with this drug.
Neratinib (*Nerlynx*) Puma	Neratinib is a kinase inhibitor that irreversibly binds to epidermal growth factor receptor (EGFR), human epidermal growth factor receptor 2 (HER2), and HER4. Neratinib is an adjuvant treatment of adult patients with early-stage HER2−overexpressed/amplified breast cancer, to follow adjuvant trastuzumab-based therapy.

Drug Name Generic (Brand), Maker	Actions/Common Side Effects*
Palbociclib (*Ibrance*) Pfizer	Palbociclib inhibits cyclin-dependent kinases 4 and 6 (CDK4 and CDK6). It is used to treat women or men with HR+/HER2– advanced or metastatic breast cancer in combination with an aromatase inhibitor as initial endocrine-based therapy in post-menopausal women or in men or with fulvestrant in patients whose cancer has progressed following endocrine therapy. Key side effects include low white blood cell counts and interstitial lung disease/pneumonitis.
Ribociclib (*Kisqali*) Novartis	Ribociclib inhibits cyclin-dependent kinases 4 and 6 (CDK4 and CDK6). It is used to treat women or men with HR+/HER2– advanced or metastatic breast cancer in combination with an aromatase inhibitor as initial endocrine-based therapy in post-menopausal women or in men or with fulvestrant in patients whose cancer has progressed following endocrine therapy.
PARP INHIBITORS	**Medications used to improve the ability of standard chemotherapy drugs to kill cancer cells.**
Olaparib (*Lynparza*) AstraZeneca	Olaparib is an inhibitor of poly (ADP-ribose) poly-merase (PARP) enzymes, including PARP1, PARP2, and PARP3. PARP enzymes are involved in normal cellular functions, such as DNA transcription and DNA repair. It is used in patients with deleterious or suspected deleterious germline *BRCA*-mutated (gBRCAm) advanced breast cancer who have been treated with three or more prior lines of chemother-apy. Patients are identified as potential candidates for therapy based on an FDA-approved companion diagnostics. Potential side effects include pneumo-nitis and myelodysplastic syndrome or acute myeloid leukemia.

(Continues)

Table 1 Drugs Used in the Treatment of Breast Cancer (*Continued*)

Drug Name Generic (Brand), Maker	Actions/Common Side Effects*
Talazoparib (*Talzenna*) Pfizer	Talazoparib is an inhibitor of poly (ADP-ribose) polymerase (PARP) enzymes, including PARP1, PARP2, and PARP3. PARP enzymes are involved in normal cellular functions, such as DNA transcription and DNA repair. It is used in patients with deleterious or suspected deleterious germline *BRCA*-mutated (gBRCAm) HER2– advanced breast cancer identified as candidates by an FDA-approved diagnostic test. Potential long-term side effects include myelosuppression and myelodysplastic syndrome or acute myeloid leukemia.

*Drug information has been drawn from *The Physicians' Desk Reference*, the FDA website, CancerSource.com Drug Guide, and, in some cases, specific pharmaceutical companies' websites. Not all known side effects are listed here; consult with your doctor if you are experiencing side effects, whether they are listed here or not. Many of these medications also have interactions with other medications that produce symptoms not listed here.

Table 2 Hormonal Therapies Used in Breast Cancer Treatment*

Drug Name Generic (Brand), Maker	Type/Effects	Used for
Anastrozole (*Arimidex*) AstraZeneca Pharmaceuticals	Aromatase inhibitor (reversible); prevents production of estrogen in adrenal glands	Initial adjuvant treatment of postmenopausal women with hormone receptor-positive breast cancer.
Exemestane (*Aromasin*) Pfizer	Aromatase inhibitor (irreversible)	Adjuvant treatment of advanced breast cancer in postmenopausal women who have received 2–3 years of tamoxifen and are switched to exemestane to complete the 5 years of tamoxifen therapy.
Fulvestrant injection (*Faslodex*) AstraZeneca Pharmaceuticals	Estrogen receptor antagonist	Treatment of hormone receptor-positive metastatic breast cancer in postmenopausal women with disease progression following anti-estrogen therapy. Recent research has confirmed that taking a higher dosage (500 mg) of this hormonal therapy than previously used improves the clinical outcomes

Drug Name Generic (Brand), Maker	Type/Effects	Used for
		slowing or stopping the progression of the disease. If on a lower dosage (250 mg), ask your medical oncologist if you are a candidate to take this medication in the future at the new FDA-approved dosage of 500 mg.
Goserelin (*Zoladex*)	GnRH agonist	Approved for premenopausal and perimeno-pausal women with advanced HR+ breast cancer. For women at high risk of recurrence, this treatment offers significantly more endocrine suppression than oophorectomy, allowing younger women with cancer the option of receiv-ing cancer treatment while potentially salvaging future fertility. Side effects include hyperglycemia and risk of developing or worsening diabetes, injection site reactions, increased risk of cardio-vascular disease, and electrolyte abnormalities.
Letrozole (*Femara*) Novartis Pharmaceuticals		Adjuvant treatment of postmenopausal women with hormone receptor-positive early breast cancer. The effectiveness of letrozole in early breast cancer is based on an analysis of disease-free survival in patients treated for a median of 24 months and followed for a median of 26 months. Follow-up analyses will determine long-term outcomes for both safety and efficacy. Letrozole is also used for the extended adjuvant treatment of early breast cancer in postmeno-pausal women who have received 5 years of adjuvant tamoxifen therapy. The effectiveness of letrozole in extended adjuvant treatment of early breast cancer is based on an analysis of dis-ease-free survival in patients treated for a me-dian of 24 months. Further data will be required to determine long-term outcome. Letrozole is also used for first-line treatment of postmeno-pausal women with hormone receptor-positive or hormone receptor-unknown locally advanced or metastatic breast cancer.

(Continues)

Table 2 Hormonal Therapies Used in Breast Cancer Treatment* (*Continued*)

Drug Name Generic (Brand), Maker	Type/Effects	Used for
	Aromatase inhibitor (reversible)	Letrozole is also indicated for the treatment of advanced breast cancer in postmenopausal women with disease progression following anti-estrogen therapy.
Megestrol acetate (*Megace*) Bristol-Myers Squibb	Aromatase inhibitor; mimics action of progesterone, blocking it from progesterone receptors	An older drug previously used to treat PR+ cancers. Because it is also an appetite stimulant, it may be preferred for underweight patients who have responsive cancers, but it is generally rarely used in treating cancer except in limited circumstances.
Tamoxifen citrate (*Nolvadex*) AstraZeneca	Binds to estrogen receptors, blocking estrogen from the cancer cells	Tamoxifen is effective in the treatment of metastatic breast cancer in women and men. In premenopausal women with metastatic breast cancer, tamoxifen offers an alternative to oophorectomy or ovarian irradiation. Patients whose tumors are estrogen receptor positive are more likely to benefit from tamoxifen. It is used for treating breast cancer in postmenopausal women following total mastectomy or segmental mastectomy, axillary dissection, and breast irradiation. It also reduces the occurrence of contralateral breast cancer in patients receiving adjuvant therapy with tamoxifen citrate for breast cancer. In women with DCIS, following breast surgery and radiation, tamoxifen is used to reduce the risk of invasive breast cancer. It is also used to reduce the incidence of breast cancer in women at high risk for breast cancer, defined as women at least 35 years of age with a 5-year predicted risk of breast cancer.
Toremifene citrate (*Fareston*) Orion Corporation	Aromatase inhibitor	Treatment of metastatic breast cancer in postmenopausal women with ER+ or receptor-unknown tumors.

*Drug information has been drawn from *The Physicians' Desk Reference*, the FDA website, CancerSource.com Drug Guide, and, in some cases, specific pharmaceutical companies' websites. Not all known side effects are listed here; consult with your doctor if you are experiencing side effects, whether they are listed here or not. Many of these medications also have interactions with other medications that produce symptoms not listed here.

Appendix

Resources to Benefit Metastatic Breast Cancer Patients and Their Families

American Cancer Society
(800) ACS-2345
https://www.cancer.org/content/cancer/en/search.html?q=metastatic+breast+cancer

American Society of Clinical Oncology (ASCO)
American Society of Clinical Oncology
1900 Duke Street, Suite 200
Alexandria, VA 22314
(703) 299-0150
Email: asco@asco.org
www.asco.org

Breastcancer.org
(610) 642-6550
Email: comments@breastcancer.org
www.breastcancer.org

Cancer Care, Inc.
(800) 813-HOPE
Email: info@cancercare.org
www.cancercare.org

Cancer Research Institute
(800) 99-CANCER
www.cancerresearch.org

CenterWatch Clinical Trials Listing Service
22 Thomson Place, 47F1
Boston, MA 02210-1212
(617) 856-5900
www.centerwatch.com/patient/trials.html

Financial Planning Association
1600 K Street NW
Washington, DC 20006
(800) 282-75296
www.fpanet.org

The Johns Hopkins Breast Center
www.hopkinsmedicine.org/breast_center

Living Beyond Breast Cancer
354 W. Lancaster Avenue, Suite 224
Haverford, PA 19041
National Helpline
(888) 753-5222
(484) 708-1550
Email: mail@lbbc.org
www.lbbc.org

Metastatic Breast Cancer Network
mbcn.org
(888) 500-0370
Email: mbcn@mbcn.org

Metavivor
(818) 860-1226
www.metavivor.org

Mothers Supporting Daughters with Breast Cancer (MSDBC)
(410) 778-1982
Email: msdbc@verizon.net
www.mothersdaughters.org

National Breast Cancer Coalition
1101 17th Street NW, Suite 1300
Washington, DC 20036
(800) 622-2838
(202) 265-6854
www.StopBreastCancer.org

National Cancer Institute
Public Office of Information
Building 31, Room 10A31
31 Center Drive, MSC 2580
Bethesda, MD 20892-2580
(800) 4-CANCER
www.cancer.gov

National Center for Complementary and Alternative Medicine
(888) 644-6226
Email: info@nccam.nih.gov
www.nccam.nih.gov

National Comprehensive Cancer Network
(888) 909-NCCN
www.nccn.org

National Institutes of Health
National Institutes of Health
9000 Rockville Pike
Bethesda, Maryland 20892
(301) 496-4000
NIHInfo@do.nih.gov
www.nih.gov
www.clinicaltrials.gov (for information on clinical trials)

National Metastatic Breast Cancer Alliance
https://www.mbcalliance.org/
https://www.mbcalliance.org/support

The Story Half Told
produced by Pfizer
https://www.storyhalftold.com/

Susan G. Komen for the Cure
National Helpline
   (800) IM-AWARE
www.breastcancerinfo.com

Y-ME
(800) 221-2141
   (24-hour national hotline)
(800) 986-9505
   (24-hour hotline in Spanish)
Email: info@y-me.org
www.y-me.org

Young Survival Coalition
61 Broadway, Suite 2235
New York, NY 10006
(877) YSC-1011
(646) 257-3000
Email: info@youngsurvival.org
www.youngsurvival.org

Where can I get help with financial or legal concerns?

Accompanying any serious illness are questions and concerns related to expenses incurred as a result of treatment, health insurance questions that can be overwhelming to try to understand or resolve alone, and sometimes even legal questions related to employment or financial matters. This list of national resources can aid you in addressing your concerns. However, also take the time to meet with your social worker and patient navigator who will have access to local resources for you in the form of advocacy organizations that provide financial support to breast cancer patients to help with household bills, prescription costs, and other financial needs. These individuals will also know how to obtain discounted drugs from the pharmaceutical companies that manufacture some of the treatments you may be taking. There are also pro bono (work for free) lawyers within all local communities to help patients like you with legal matters that need to be addressed.

America's Health Insurance Plans
601 Pennsylvania Avenue NW, South Bldg., Suite 500
Washington, DC 20004
(202) 778-3200
Email: ahip@ahip.org
www.ahip.org

Cancer Care, Inc.
(800) 813-HOPE
Email: info@cancercare.org
www.cancercare.org

Credit Counseling Centers of America/Money Management International
(800) 493-2222
www.cccamerica.org

National Association of Hospital Hospitality Houses, Inc.
PO Box 18087
Asheville, NC 22814-0087
(800) 542-9730
(828) 253-1188
Email: helpinghomes@nahhh.org
www.nahhh.org

National Coalition for Cancer Survivorship (NCCS)
1010 Wayne Avenue, Suite 770
Silver Spring, MD 20910
(888) 650-9127
(301) 650-9127
Email: info@ccansearch.org
www.canceradvocacy.org

Patient Advocate Foundation
700 Thimble Shoals Boulevard, Suite 200
Newport News, VA 23606
(800) 532-5274
(757) 873-6668
Email: help@patientadvocate.org
www.patientadvocate.org

Social Security Administration
Office of Public Inquiries
(800) 772-1213
www.ssa.gov

Glossary

A

Ablation: A nonsurgical technique for destroying cancerous tissue using heat or cold delivered directly to the tumor site.

Acupuncture: The technique of inserting thin needles into the skin at specific points. This can help control pain and other symptoms for some individuals and is a form of ancient Chinese medicine. It is a form of complementary therapy.

Adjuncts: A treatment that complements another treatment.

Adjuvant therapy: Treatment given after the primary treatment to increase the chances of a cure, and treatment to prevent the cancer from recurring.

Adjuvant studies: A clinical trial to determine if additional therapy will further opportunity for survival.

Advance directives: Legal documents that allow people to express their decisions regarding what they do and don't want to have done during their last weeks or months in case they become unable to communicate effectively.

Agent: A specific chemical that can be used alone or in combination with another agent to treat cancer.

Alopecia: Hair loss.

Alternative medicine: Medicines used in lieu of standard medical therapies.

Analgesic: Drugs that reduce pain.

Anemia: A condition in which the number of red blood cells is too low.

Antibodies: Special proteins produced by your immune system. They help protect the body from disease.

Anti-estrogen drug: A drug that suppresses estrogen and damages the estrogen receptor but has no estrogen agonist effects.

Antigens: Specific cells that substances that are not supposed to be in your body (like viruses, bacteria, or cell changes that are very abnormal) produce.

Antiemetics: Drugs to stop or prevent nausea or vomiting.

Aromatase inhibitor: Drugs that lower the amount of estrogen made in the body after menopause. This can slow or stop the growth of cancer that needs estrogen to grow.

Ascites: A buildup of fluid in the abdominal cavity.

Asymptomatic: Not manifesting any symptoms.

B

Biological pathways: The complex interactions among hormones and proteins within a cell that cause changes in the cell's behavior.

Biopsy: A procedure in which cells are collected for microscopic examination.

Bone density (DEXA) scan: A test to evaluate bone mineral density. The results predict the likelihood of fracture. The DEXA scan calculates bone density based on the amount of radiation absorbed by the bone and compares your bone strength with that of young premenopausal women.

Bone scan: An X-ray that looks for signs of metastasis to the bones.

Breast cancer case conference: Same as tumor board. A special meeting of oncology doctors and nurses for the purpose of discussing a specific patient's case and planning a recommended treatment. Usually involves the review of pathology slides, mammograms, other X-rays, and a discussion about what would be the best course of action for treating the patient's breast cancer.

Breast cancer tumor board: Same as case conference. A special meeting of oncology doctors and nurses for the purpose of discussing a specific patient's case and planning a recommended treatment. Usually involves the review of pathology slides, mammograms, other X-rays, and a discussion about what would be the best course of action for treating the patient's breast cancer.

Breast mass: An abnormal collection of tissue within the breast.

C

Cancer: The presence of malignant cells.

CDK4/6 inhibitors: A class of drugs that target enzymes called CDK4 and CDK6 that are important in cell division. CDK4/6 inhibitors are designed to interrupt the growth of cancer cells.

Cells: Basic elements of tissues; the appearance and composition of individual cells are unique to the tissue they compose.

Chemotherapy: Treatment with drugs that kill cancer cells or make them less active. It is a form of systemic treatment.

Clinical trials: Research studies in which patients are offered the opportunity to try new innovative therapies (under careful observation) in order to help doctors identify the best treatments with the fewest side effects. These studies help improve the overall standard of care.

Combination therapy: Treatment using more than one type of therapy at a time.

Complementary and alternative medicine (CAM): Forms of treatment that are used in addition to, or instead of, standard treatments. Their purpose is to strengthen your whole mind and body to maximize your health, energy, and well-being. These practices are not considered "standard" medical approaches. They include dietary supplements, vitamins, herbal preparations, special teas, massage therapy, acupuncture, spiritual healing, visualization, and meditation.

Complementary therapy: Medicines used in conjunction with standard therapies.

Cryoablation: A tumor ablation method that delivers cold gas to a tumor in order to kill cancer cells by freezing them.

Cytopenia: Low cell count (usually in relation to white blood cells).

Cytotoxic: A term used to describe anything that kills cells.

D

Distant recurrence: The breast cancer has been found now in another organ, such as the lungs, liver, bones, or brain. It is located outside of the breast and lymph nodes near the breast.

E

Echocardiogram: A special test using ultrasound that determines the strength of the heart.

Estrogen: Female hormone related to childbearing.

Estrogen receptor-positive cancer: A cancer that grows more rapidly with exposure to the hormone estrogen.

F

First-line therapy: The first drug or set of drugs that you receive as your treatment.

Fluorescence in situ hybridization (FISH): This is a lab test that measures the amount of a certain gene in cells. It can be used to see if an invasive cancer has too many HER2 genes. A cancer with too many of these genes is called HER2–positive.

G

Guided imagery: A mind–body technique in which the patient visualizes and meditates upon images that encourage a positive immune response.

H

Healthcare proxy: A designated person authorized by you to make decisions regarding your medical treatment when you are unable to do so.

Hemoglobin: The part of the red blood cell that carries the oxygen.

HER2 overexpression: An excess of a certain protein (HER2) on the surface of a cell that may be related to a high number of abnormal or defective cells.

Hormonal therapy: Treatment that blocks the effects of hormones upon cancers that depend on hormones to grow (also referred to as endocrine therapy).

Hormone: Chemical messengers in the body.

Hormone receptor: A protein on the surface or inside a cell that connects to a certain hormone (estrogen or progesterone) and causes changes in the cell.

Hormone replacement therapy: Administration of artificial estrogen and progesterone to alleviate the symptoms of menopause and to prevent health problems experienced by postmenopausal women, particularly osteoporosis.

Hospice: An organization that provides programs and services designed to help alleviate the physical and psychosocial suffering associated with progressive incurable illness.

Hypercalcemia: Accelerated loss of calcium in bones, leading to elevated levels of the mineral in the bloodstream with symptoms such as nausea and confusion.

I

Immune checkpoint: A connection between the PD-1 protein on T cells and PD-L1 protein on cancer cells that causes the immune system to ignore the cancerous cell rather than kill it.

Immunohistochemistry (IHC): The most commonly used test to see if a tumor has too much of the HER2–receptor protein on the surface of the cancer cells. The IHC test gives a score of 0 to 31 that indicates the amount of HER2–receptor protein. It also measures the presence of hormone receptors on the breast cancer cell and determines if a tumor is hormone receptor-positive or -negative.

Implantable port: A disk placed under the skin to allow repeated direct access into a blood vessel.

Incidence: The number of times a disease occurs within a population of people.

K

Ki67: A molecule that can be easily detected in growing cells in order to gain an understanding of the rate at which the cells within a tumor are growing.

L

Living will: Outlines what care you want in the event you become unable to communicate due to coma or heavy sedation.

Locally advanced disease: Stage III breast cancer. Cancer that is in a large area of the breast and lymph nodes under the arm; it may be fixed on the chest wall.

Local recurrence: The breast cancer has returned inside the breast after treatment was completed.

Local treatment: Refers to anything that is targeted to a specific area of the body—such as the breast, the lymph nodes, the lungs—as opposed to the whole body.

Lumpectomy: Breast cancer surgery to remove the breast cancer and a small amount of normal tissue surrounding it.

Lymph: Fluid carried through the body by the lymphatic system, composed primarily of white blood cells and diluted plasma.

Lymph nodes: Tissues in the lymphatic system that filter lymph fluid and help the immune system fight disease.

M

Malignant: Cancerous; growing rapidly and out of control.

Mastectomy: Surgery that removes the whole breast.

Medical oncologist: See oncologist.

Meditation: A mental technique that clears the mind and relaxes the body through concentration.

Menopause: End of menstrual periods.

Metastasis, metastasize: The spread of cancer from one part of the body to another.

Metastatic breast cancer: Cancer that has spread from the breast to other organ sites such as the liver, lung, bone, or brain.

Micrometastases: Small numbers of cancer cells that have spread from the primary tumor to other parts of the body and are too few to be picked up in a screening or diagnostic test.

Microwave ablation: A tumor ablation method that relies on microwaves to create heat energy to destroy cancer cells.

Monoclonal antibody: Medications that target antigens in specific cell types or tissues.

Mucositis: A condition in which the mucosa (the lining of the digestive tract, from the mouth to the anus) becomes swollen, red, and sore. For example, sores in the mouth that can be a side effect of chemotherapy.

MUGA test: A special test that determines the strength of the heart and is given for women having chemotherapy or targeted therapy that may cause heart problems as a complication.

Mutation: A change or error in a gene. Specific mutations have been linked with breast cancer.

N

Nadir: The low point of blood counts that occurs as a result of chemotherapy.

National Comprehensive Cancer Network (NCCN): An organization composed of specific cancer centers across the country that excel in cancer diagnosis and treatment that work together to create treatment guidelines followed no matter where patients are receiving their care.

NED: No evidence of disease on scans.

Nerve blocks: An anesthetic injection that stops nerve impulses for pain relief.

Neutropenia: An abnormally low number of a particular type of white blood cell called a neutrophil. White blood cells (leukocytes) are the cells in the blood that play important roles by fighting off infection.

Neutropenic fever: A fever due to a low white blood cell count, usually caused by a side effect of chemotherapy.

Noninvasive cancer: Cancer confined to its tissue point of origin and not found in surrounding tissues.

Nonsteroidal anti-inflammatory drugs (NSAIDs): A class of pain medications, often sold over the counter, that includes ibuprofen and similar common painkillers.

Nurse navigator: A healthcare professional who helps patients in navigating their care and treatment by assisting them with scheduling appointments, answering questions related to test results, patient education, support, and providing guidance in decision making across the continuum of care.

O

Oncogene: A mutated form of a gene that normally regulates cell growth, which under certain conditions can cause cancer. HER2 is an oncogene of human epidermal growth factor receptor.

Oncologist: A cancer specialist who helps determine treatment choices.

Oophorectomy: An operation to remove the ovaries.

Osteonecrosis: When some noncancerous bone cells die off in a way that is not normal.

Osteopenia: A condition of less bone density or bone mass than would be normally expected if you compare a woman to a woman or population of women her age. It is the bone loss that, if it continues, can lead to osteoporosis.

Ovarian ablation: Using surgery or radiation to reduce or eliminate the ovaries' ability to produce estrogen.

Overall survival: The percentage of people in a study who have survived for a certain period of time, usually reported as time since diagnosis or treatment. Often called the survival rate.

P

Palliative care: Care to relieve the symptoms of cancer and to keep the best quality of life for as long as possible without seeking to cure cancer.

Paracentesis: A procedure to take out fluid that has collected in the abdominal cavity. This fluid buildup, called ascites, may be caused by infection, inflammation, an injury, or other conditions, such as cancer. The fluid is taken out using a long thin needle put through the belly. The fluid is sent to a lab and studied to find the cause of the fluid buildup. Paracentesis also may be done to take the fluid out to relieve belly pressure or pain in people with cancer or cirrhosis.

PARP inhibitors: A class of drugs that blocks an enzyme involved in tumor DNA repair (called PARP enzyme). These drugs can help chemotherapy better kill cancer cells.

Pathologist: A specialist trained to distinguish normal from abnormal cells.

PD-L1–positive breast cancer: Breast cancer that contains the PD-L1 protein, which prevents immune cells from killing the cancer.

Pedigree: A family tree that documents different kinds of cancers occurring within your family, usually three generations back.

Peripheral neuropathy: Numbness and pain of the hands and feet, which can be caused by infection, very strong drugs (such as chemotherapy), or disease.

Phases: A series of steps followed in clinical trials.

Placebo: A pill or treatment that looks the same and is taken in the same way as a drug or treatment in a clinical trial but contains no active drug ingredients.

Platelets: Components of blood that assist in clotting and wound healing.

Pleural cavity: A space between the outside of the lungs and the inside wall of the chest cavity.

Pleural effusion: Excess fluid that accumulates in the pleural cavity, the fluid-filled space that surrounds the lungs. This excess fluid can impair breathing by limiting the expansion of the lungs.

Pleurodesis: A procedure that gets rid of the open space between the lung and the chest cavity. This is done to stop fluid from building up in this space. When cancer cells are growing in this space, they make fluid that can collect and cause difficulty breathing. During this surgery, a chemical is placed in the space. Your body's reaction to the chemical causes the lining around the lung to stick to the inside lining of the chest wall.

Port: The treatment site.

Primary care provider (PCP): The patient's normal healthcare provider, usually an internal medicine or family medicine practitioner.

Progesterone: A female hormone that regulates the menstrual cycle and is crucial for pregnancy.

Progesterone receptor-positive cancer: Cancer that grows more rapidly with exposure to the hormone progesterone.

Prognosis: An estimation of the likely outcome of an illness based upon the patient's current status and the available treatments.

Prognostic factors: Identifiable features of the cancer that help determine how best to treat it and what its long-term prognosis may be.

Progression-free survival: The length of time during and after treatment in which a patient is living with a disease that does not get worse. Progression-free survival may be used in a clinical study or trial to help find out how well a new treatment works.

Protocols: The research plan for how the drug is given and to whom it is given.

Pulmonary embolism: Blockage of blood vessels in the lungs that interfere with breathing.

Q

Quality of life: The aspects of life that make it enjoyable and worth living. Cancer treatment balances the need to keep the body alive against whether the life is of acceptable quality.

R

Radiofrequency ablation: A tumor ablation method that relies on radio waves to create heat energy to destroy cancer cells.

Radiologist: A physician who specializes in radiology, which includes reading of X-rays, scans, and other imaging studies used to diagnose various conditions and diseases.

Radiation oncologist: A cancer specialist who determines the amount of radiotherapy required.

Radiation physicist: A specialist who makes sure that radiotherapy equipment is working properly and that the machines deliver the right dose of radiation.

Radiation therapy: The use of high-energy X-rays to kill cancer cells and shrink tumors.

Randomized: Describes the process in a clinical trial in which animal or human subjects are assigned by chance to separate groups that allow for comparison of different treatments.

Recurrent cancer: The disease has come back in spite of the initial treatment.

Red blood cells (RBCs): Cells in the blood with the primary function of carrying oxygen to tissues.

Remission: A decrease in or disappearance of signs and symptoms of cancer. In partial remission, some, but not all, signs and symptoms have disappeared. In complete remission, all signs and symptoms have disappeared, although there may still be cancer cells present in the body.

Risk factors: Any factors that contribute to an increased possibility of getting cancer.

S

Scans: Techniques to create images of specific parts of the body on a computer screen or on film.

Selective estrogen receptor modulators (SERMs): Drugs that bind to the estrogen receptor. In some tissues (breast), SERMs act as estrogen antagonists; in others, they act as estrogen agonists.

Stage: A numerical determination of how far the cancer has progressed.

Standard of care: A diagnostic and treatment process that a clinician should follow for a certain type of patient, illness, or clinical circumstances.

Surgical oncologist: A specialist trained in surgical removal of cancerous tumors.

Systemic treatment: A treatment that affects the whole body (the patient's whole system).

T

Targeted biologic therapy: Cancer treatments that target specific characteristics of cancer cells, such as a protein, an enzyme, or the formation of new blood vessels. Targeted therapies don't harm healthy normal cells.

Thoracentesis: The removal of fluid from the pleural cavity through a hollow needle inserted between the ribs.

Total (simple) mastectomy: When a surgeon removes the whole breast but does not remove lymph nodes.

Tumor: A mass or lump of extra tissue.

U

Ultrasound: Uses sound waves to determine whether a lump is solid or filled with fluid.

Uterine cancer: A cancer beginning in the uterus; sometimes related genetically to breast cancer.

V

Vascular access device (VAD): A special catheter is inserted inside a major vein (generally in one of the large veins in the neck) extending into the large central vein near the heart so that blood can be repeatedly drawn or medication and nutrients can be injected into the patient's bloodstream on a continual basis or dialysis can be performed.

Vascular endothelial growth factor (VEGF): A substance made by cells that causes new blood vessels to form.

Vertebroplasty: A procedure to relieve pain from fractures of the vertebrae, in which a special cement is injected into the fractured bone.

Index